John S. Wodarski, PhD
Marvin D. Feit, PhD

Adolescent Substance Abuse: An Empirical-Based Group Preventive Health Paradigm

Pre-publication
REVIEW

"**T**his is a practical instructional text that has implications for a wide audience of educators, health care professionals, and counselors in a variety of fields of practice—schools, drop-in centers, health and mental health settings, correctional rehabilitation settings, and social welfare institutions. The material has broad appeal to any setting that touches the lives of adolescents.

The authors appropriately square the issue of substance abuse where it belongs: with adolescents themselves and with their families. They present in detail the curriculums of the Teams-Games-Tournaments approach and the Comprehensive Psychoactive Substance Abuse Education Program, both of which have proven successful with these populations.

The comprehensiveness of these programs is easy to read, clear, rich in examples, and presented in a simplified step-by-step fashion. This is the overall strength of the text. Drs. Wodarski and Feit do not tout their approach as the 'be all and end all' but as something that works for a very real social problem."

Michael J. Holosko, PhD
Professor of Social Work,
University of Windsor,
Ontario, Canada

Adolescent Substance Abuse
An Empirical-Based Group Preventive Health Paradigm

HAWORTH Health and Social Policy
Marvin D. Feit, PhD
Senior Editor

New, Recent, and Forthcoming Titles:

Maltreatment and the School-Age Child: Developmental Outcomes and System Issues by Phyllis T. Howing, John S. Wodarski, P. David Kurtz, and James Martin Gaudin, Jr.

Health and Social Policy edited by Marvin D. Feit and Stanley F. Battle

Adolescent Substance Abuse: An Empirical-Based Group Preventive Health Paradigm by John S. Wodarski and Marvin D. Feit

Adolescent Substance Abuse
An Empirical-Based Group Preventive Health Paradigm

John S. Wodarski, PhD
Marvin D. Feit, PhD

The Haworth Press
New York • London

The Haworth Press, Inc., 10 Alice Street, Binghamton, NY 13904-1580

Library of Congress Cataloging-in-Publication Data

Wodarski, John S.
    Adolescent substance abuse : an empirical-based group preventive health paradigm / John S. Wodarski, Marvin D. Feit.
       p.   cm.
    Includes bibliographical references and index.
    ISBN 1-56024-880-7 (acid-free paper)
    1. Teenagers–Substance use. 2. Substance abuse–Prevention. 3. Substance abuse–Study and teaching. I. Feit, Marvin D. II. Title.
RJ506.D78W635 1995   94-29995
362.29'17'0835–dc20   CIP

CONTENTS

ABOUT THE AUTHORS

John S. Wodarski, PhD, is Janet B. Wattles Professor and Director of the Doctoral Program and Research Center at the State University of New York at Buffalo. Among the top scholars in social work, he has authored or co-authored nearly 200 publications, including 17 books. Dr. Wodarski has a reputation as an excellent teacher and won a Social Work Professor of the Year award at the University of Georgia in 1988. His strengths are in child welfare and alcohol-based problems and his commitment to empirically based practice.

Marvin D. Feit, PhD, is Professor and Director of the School of Social Work at the University of Akron, Ohio. The author or co-author of several books, he has written many articles and chapters in the areas of group work, substance abuse, health, and practice. He has made numerous presentations at national, state, and local conferences, and has served as a consultant to profit and nonprofit organizations, federal and state government agencies, and numerous community-based agencies. Dr. Feit is a founding editor of the *Journal of Health & Social Policy.*

Preface

People of all ages are dying from substance abuse at an alarming rate. In spite of the magnitude of the problem, however, there is concern that society's attitude toward drugs is one of ambivalence (Nobel, Maxwell, and West, 1984). Macrosystem changes are needed to reorient society to the dangers of its complacency. Substance abuse is a problem for all age groups as well as the social system in its entirety. The individual, his or her peer group, family (both nuclear and extended), school, and community at large are all affected by the escapades of even one substance-abusing person.

Substance abuse is frequently either the cause or the effect of stress experienced during adolescence (Hamburg and Petersen, 1986). Because school, peers, and family are the primary influences in an adolescent's life, preventative programs should focus on these areas to increase their prosocial influences.

Attempts to reverse the trend of acceptance of substance abuse have been characterized by their focus on only certain aspects of the problem. This singular focus has resulted in the limited effectiveness of prevention programs (Johnson, 1984; Wodarski and Hoffman, 1984).

With multiple forces influencing adolescents and resulting in substance abuse, macrolevel change in societal norms and values regarding substance abuse is necessary. There are a number of agents of change that can be effective: development of appropriate treatment paradigms, family intervention, school and peer-group environments, the teams-games-tournaments program, the media, community movements, law enforcement, and business and industry.

The solution to the problem of substance abuse requires an all-out effort by those societal forces capable of effecting change. Families, schools, peers, communities, businesses, and the media all must share the responsibility both for previously condoning actions that have perpetuated the problem and for working toward mutual goals and solutions in the future; they all possess the power to help eradicate this social problem. The campaign cannot be waged on one front; combined, cooperative efforts are essential. This text is devoted to helping practitioners reduce the significant costs of adolescent substance abuse.

John S. Wodarski
Marvin Feit

REFERENCES

Johnson, N. (1984). Research Reports: Reducing Community Alcohol Problems. *Alcohol Health World,* 8, 60-61.

Hamburg, B.A. and Peterson, A.C. (1986). Adolescence: A Developmental Approach to Problems and Psychopathology. *Behavioral Therapy,* 17, 480-499.

Nobel, E.P., Maxwell, D.S., and West, L.J. (1984). Alcoholism. *American Internal Medicine,* 100, 405-416.

Wodarski, J.S. and Hoffman, S.D. (1984). Alcohol Education for Adolescents. *Social Work Education,* 6, 69-92.

Chapter 1

Adolescent Substance Abuse:
An Introduction

America today is a chemical culture (Morrison, 1985). An estimated 18 million adults 18 years and older in the United States currently experience problems as a result of alcohol use. Of these, 10.6 million suffer from the disease of alcoholism. Alcohol-related problems may include symptoms of alcohol dependence such as memory loss, inability to stop drinking until intoxicated, inability to cut down on drinking, binge drinking, and withdrawal symptoms.

Seventy million Americans, or 37 percent of the total U.S. population aged 12 and above, have used marijuana, cocaine, or another illicit drug at some time in their lives according to National Household Survey of Drug Abuse (National Institute on Drug Abuse, 1985). Of these 23 million, or 12 percent, were "current" users, i.e., they had used an illegal drug within the last 30 days. The use of marijuana and other drugs had declined since the comparable 1982 survey, although cocaine use increased.

The use and abuse of chemical substances exacts an incalculable cost for substance abusers and nonsubstance abusers alike. Alcohol abuse and alcoholism cost the United States $116.8 billion in 1983. Costs due to premature death were $18 billion. Yet, drug abuse-related deaths, injury, disease, and family and emotional disturbance are consequences that cannot be measured in monetary figures. Annually, 100,000 to 120,000 deaths are directly attributable to substance abuse, and another 120,000 to 150,000 deaths are substance abuse related.

Alcohol is a factor in nearly half of all accidental deaths, suicides, and homicides, including 42 percent of all deaths from motor vehicle accidents. Of increasing concern is the role of drug use in the transmission of HIV. The intravenous drug-user population (including homosexual intravenous drug users) accounts for 25 percent of all AIDS patients. The disease is contracted through sexual transmission and the sharing of contaminated needles among this group (National Institute on Drug Abuse, 1985).

The abuse of alcohol and other drugs among our youth is a problem of alarming scope and gravity. According to the American Medical Association (1991) in 1988, 6 percent of 12 to 17 year olds consumed alcohol daily, 4 percent used marijuana daily, and 0.5 percent used cocaine daily. Morrison (1985) notes that two-thirds of high school students use drugs and alcohol with regular frequency, and 85 percent of these students use drugs and alcohol at least three times a week. Additionally, 65 percent to 70 percent of junior high school students use drugs and alcohol two to three times weekly.

Findings from the University of Michigan's Institute for Social Research's multi-year Monitoring the Future surveys ("Patterns of Drug Use," 1987-1988) continue to tell a troubling story of drug use among young people nationwide. Responses to the 1987 survey indicate that over half of last year's high school seniors (57 percent) had tried an illicit drug, and over one-third (36 percent) had tried an illicit drug other than marijuana. One in every six or seven high school seniors had tried cocaine (15.2 percent) and one in 18 (5.6 percent) had tried "crack"–the especially risky form of cocaine. The study also reveals that by age 27, 40 percent of young adults have had some experience with cocaine. Two other classes of drugs–alcohol and cigarettes–have remained overwhelmingly popular among young people. Nearly all of 1987's high school seniors (92 percent) reported some experience with alcohol, and nearly 40 percent reported having had five or more drinks in a row in the two weeks just prior to the survey.

Adolescence has been identified as a time when experimentation with drugs may be most active (Mayer & Filstead, 1980). The acute consequences of substance use and misuse include traffic accidents, death due to accidents, later life health problems, suicide, school-related problems, temporary sickness, and absenteeism (Barr, Antes, Ottenberg, & Rosen, 1984). One-fourth of all alcohol and drug-related motor vehicle fatalities involve males age 16 to 19 (Morrison 1985). Drug overdoses result in 88 percent of all adolescent suicides, and more teenagers die in alcohol and drug-related motor vehicle accidents than from any disease (Morrison, 1985).

The cost of drinking and subsequent driving among teenagers presents a significant social problem in this country. In 1980 alone there were 1,289,443 persons arrested for driving while under the influence of alcohol. Of those, 29,957 were under the age of 18 and 696 were under age 15! And there appears to be a trend toward a progressively worsening situation. Arrests for DUI among those 18 and under increased 236 percent between 1971 and 1980. The outcomes of adolescent DUI are deadly. In one account, 43 percent of the approximately 50,000 persons killed in motor vehicle accidents were correlated with adolescent DUI (*Alcohol Health and Research World*, 1983). In an address at the NIAAA Alcohol and Drug Education Conference on October 4, 1982, former Health and Human Services Secretary Richard S. Schweiker stated that over 10,000 young people die in alcohol-related motor vehicle crashes each year (Allen, 1983, p. 4).

Several studies have delineated the possible consequences of adolescent substance abuse which manifest themselves in antisocial behaviors (Kane & Patterson, 1972; Mackay, 1961). Long-range consequences of teenage substance misuse include the failure to formulate goals for the future and stigmatization following an arrest while under the influence of drugs. The labeling of an adolescent under these circumstances can result in the loss of status, opportunity, and personal self-esteem (Mayer & Filstead, 1980). Patterns of substance abuse also have significant health consequences (Elliott, Huizinga & Menard, 1989; Prendergast & Schafer, 1974).

Substance use by teens takes its toll in other ways, also. The drug-abusing teen may feel isolated from nonabusing peers. Crime may become a factor to deal with when the adolescent has to steal to maintain drug habits. There are also developmental issues to be recognized. Adolescents already dealing with stressful changes in their lives may compound the stress with drug use. They are changing in physical, emotional, and sexual ways and must deal with new roles, feelings, and identities (Kandel, Simcha-Fagan, & Davies, 1986).

The issue is further compounded by multiple abuse patterns. Young people frequently use alcohol in combination with other drugs, principally marijuana (Lowman, Hubbard, Rachel, & Cavanaugh, 1982;

Turanski, 1983). This combination of alcohol and drugs adds to the difficulty in treating youths and their changing values.

Current drug users among youth (12 to 17) are also polydrug users. Of those who smoke cigarettes, 74 percent also drink alcohol, 47 percent use marijuana, and 9 percent use cocaine. Among those who drink alcohol, 37 percent also use marijuana and 5 percent use cocaine. Among those who use marijuana, 60 percent smoke cigarettes, 84 percent drink alcohol, and 12 percent use cocaine (National Institute on Drug Abuse, 1985).

The statistics bear witness to the gravity of the problem. People of all ages are dying at an alarming rate from substance abuse. Yet, society's attitude toward drugs is one of ambivalence (West, Maxwell, Noble, & Solomon, 1984). Macrosystem changes are called for in order to reorient society to the dangers of its complacency. Substance abuse is a problem for all age groups and for the total social system. The individual, his/her peer group, the family (both nuclear and extended), the school, and the community at large are all affected by the escapades of just one substance-abusing individual.

Attempts to reverse the trend of acceptance of substance abuse have been characterized by their focus on only certain aspects of the problem. This singular focus has resulted in limited effectiveness of prevention programs (Johnson, 1984; Wodarski & Hoffman, 1984).

THE NATURE OF ADOLESCENT DEVELOPMENT AND THE ROLE OF ALCOHOL AND DRUGS

Adolescence is a time of growth, stress, and change. This developmental stage affects not only the adolescent but his or her family as well. Adolescents, while in the natural process of establishing autonomy and identity, begin to separate from parents and experiment with a variety of behaviors and lifestyle patterns (Botvin, 1983). It is during adolescence when the relative importance of family and peers begins to shift. The peer group becomes more central for the adolescent, and the adolescent begins to rely more heavily on peers for support, security, and guidance. Establishing peer relationships and peer acceptance are the hallmarks of adolescence; and the need to gain acceptance, approval, and praise is greater during adolescence than at any other time in life (Morrison, 1985).

Many adolescents experience confusion and turmoil as they strive to achieve autonomy. Because of the experienced turmoil and confusion, adolescents often perceive taking psychoactive substances as one of their few pleasurable options (Morrison & Smith, 1987). According to Morrison (1985) the use and abuse of mood-altering chemical substances is now an integral part of growing into adulthood in the United States.

Substance abuse, particularly for minority youths, is frequently a part of the stress experienced, as it may be either the cause or the effect (Peterson & Hamburg, 1986). As such, it is important to develop programs to prevent substance abuse. As school, peers, and family are the primary influences on an adolescent's life, preventive programs should focus on these three areas to increase their prosocial influences.

This chapter addresses the multiple forces impacting upon adolescents and resulting in substance abuse. The aim is to propose means by which to effect macro-level change in societal norms and values regarding substance abuse. There are a number of avenues through which change can be made. This chapter will explore the following subsystems as areas of change: (1) development of appropriate treatment paradigms, (2) school and peer group environments, (3) home and family, (4) media, (5) community movements, and (6) business and industry. The second chapter describes an effective means of teaching adolescents about drugs through an empirically based teaching method called Teams, Games, and Tournaments (TGT). An effective curriculum utilizing the TGT approach is reviewed in Chapter 3. Chapter 4 contains a curriculum for parents which supports student instruction in the adolescent curriculum. The last chapter addresses issues pertinent to the reduction of adolescent substance abuse.

EFFECTIVE TREATMENT PARADIGMS

If the field of substance abuse is to progress and effective treatment and prevention paradigms are to be developed, the causal nature of substance abuse must be identified. The causal nature of substance abuse, however, is complicated and multifaceted. Most likely, each facet will require unique conceptualization of the causal chain and structuring of appropriate strategies. For example, each one of the following paradigms could be developed: substance abuse among pregnant mothers, minorities, adolescents, and so forth. Until these knowledge bases are developed, means to reduce the effects of substance abuse will be minimal (Hawkins, Abbott, Catalano, & Gillmore, 1991). The role that biological, cognitive, and learning variables play in the development and maintenance of substance abuse behaviors must be ascertained. Once this knowledge is developed, specific paradigms can be formulated according to type of client, with what type of techniques, where, and how long. Moreover, this development should include follow-up studies to ascertain the maintenance of achieved therapeutic gains (Hawkins, Lishner, Jenson, & Catalano, 1987).

A THEORETICAL PERSPECTIVE FOR THE DEVELOPMENT OF THE ADOLESCENT TREATMENT PARADIGM

Adolescence is a time when individuals become more oriented toward their peers and less toward their parents (Botvin, 1983; Bronfenbrenner, 1974; Montemayor, 1982). Adolescents turn to peers in order to receive emotional support that inattentive and unconcerned parents fail to provide. Hill (1980) stresses the importance of the conflict between parent and adolescent which leads to the adolescent accepting or seeking the approval of peers. Substantial data are available to indicate that relative to the preadolescent years, parent and adolescent perceptions of conflict increase, actual conflict increases, and effective communication decreases between parents and adolescents (e.g., Montemayor, 1982; Smith & Forehand, in press). Simultaneously, peers become increasingly influential (Montemayor, 1982). Therefore, the relative importance of family and peers must be carefully considered in adolescent drug prevention programs (Swift, 1988). Theoretical approaches to this issue range from those which view either family (Hirschi, 1969) or peers (Sutherland & Cressey, 1970) as the primary influence to those which view both family and peers as important but typically in different domains of behavior (e.g., Kandel, Kessler, & Margulies, 1978; Pentz, 1983).

Adolescence is a critical period for the development of social, cognitive, and academic skills. It is essential that we identify appropriate intervention foci to decrease substance abuse during this developmental period. At present, the best model for viewing family and peer influence on adolescent drug use is one developed by Kandel and her colleagues (e.g., Kandel, 1974a, 1980). Among other influences, the influence of parents and peers on each of the following three stages of drug use is considered: (1) initiation to hard liquor, (2) then marijuana, and finally (3) other illicit drugs. Based on a review of the available research, parents are most influential in adolescent initiation into hard liquor use and in adolescent initiation into use of illicit drugs other than marijuana, whereas peers are the primary influence in marijuana use. Parental modeling of drug use and the parental relationship with his/her adolescent are the primary mechanisms identified in adolescent drug use, whereas modeling alone appears to be the primary mechanism for peer influence.

Our theoretical perspective, as is Kandel's, is anchored within a broad base of social learning theory (Robin & Foster, 1989). From this viewpoint, the adolescent learns appropriate and inappropriate behavior from the context (that is, parents and peers) in which he/she functions by modeling and reinforcement (Bandura, 1969). That is, by observing the behaviors demonstrated by others and by receiving or not receiving reinforcement/punishment for engaging in such behaviors, adolescents acquire certain behavior patterns. Furthermore, and of particular importance, if an adolescent functions within a context in which good communication and/or adequate cognitive skills are lacking (e.g., he/she has inadequate knowledge and unrealistic beliefs, expectations, or attributions (Robin & Foster, 1989)), he/she is more likely to engage in maladaptive behavior patterns through modeling and reinforcement. Such a developmental process does not provide the adolescent with the requisite behaviors for prosocial attachment to family members, peers, and social institutions and is a high-risk factor for subsequent substance abuse.

While researchers are increasing their data base about teenage substance abuse and its consequences and are beginning to develop theoretical models of drug abuse, they know little about the effective prevention of substance misuse among teenagers. The solution to the problem of adolescent substance abuse will require an all-out effort by families, schools, peers, and communities (Fors & Rojeck, 1983; Wodarski & Fisher, 1986). However, to this point most programs have focused on only one of these variables (for reviews see Dembo & Burgos, 1976; Janvier, Guthman, & Catalano, 1980; Kinder, Pape, & Walfish, 1980; Schinke & Gilchrist, 1984).

As peers and parents are the best predictors of adolescent drug use (Adler & Kandel, 1982; Lewis & Lewis, 1984), preventive programs are needed that include one or ideally both of these groups.

If parents and peers are primary influences on adolescent drug use (e.g., Adler & Kandel, 1982; Lewis & Lewis, 1984), then prevention efforts should be directed toward developing and systematically evaluating programs with these two groups.

Data now are emerging to suggest effective procedures for dealing with peers and parents in order to prevent substance abuse. Critical questions that must be addressed are the type of interventions, their subsequent foci, and how interventions differentially affect minority, nonminority, female, and male adolescents (Hawkins, Abott, Catalano, & Gillmore, 1991).

SCHOOL AND PEER GROUP ENVIRONMENTS

Youth spend the majority of their lives in the school setting. The school system, therefore, seems to be a natural forum for implementation of change. Educational programs aimed at prevention and early intervention can negate the powerful influence of peers. An awareness of the problem of drug use among youth and recognition of ways in which society condones it are steps toward positive change. The schools can be instrumental in educating both the adolescents and their parents. Parents must be knowledgeable of the symptoms of substance abuse in adolescents. The usual signs of possible drug problems are radical changes in the usual behavioral patterns. "A definite drop in grades, bad conduct, and skipping school" are typical according to Pat Schult, senior counselor for the Young Adult Teen on the Alcohol Detoxification Unit at Peachford Hospital, Atlanta, Georgia (Okel, 1984).

Junior and senior high schools can offer parents an educational and helping network using the school as a meeting place. One school developed such a network through a parent group that initially served in an informational capacity and subsequently as a resource and support group (Turanski, 1983).

Swisher (1976) suggests that programs addressing education and prevention should include "all activities which are planned to enrich the personal development of the student . . . including humanistic education, open education, affective education, values clarification, career education and developmental guidance." This is an all-encompassing approach which needs also to be reinforced in the other areas of youths' lives.

The ideal program should have two foci. First, the information transmission approach to provide basic knowledge and awareness, and second, the responsible decision approach that will teach youngsters the basic coping and decision-making skills (Schinke, Bebel, Orlandi, & Botvin, 1988; Schinke & Gilchrist, 1984). It is important to remember that experimentation with drugs and peer pressure are related, and that peer pressure will be applied most dramatically in the school. Educators must aim to make teens more self-confident and less influenced by peer pressure. Globetti (1977) states that "in American society parents and peers are the primary socializing agencies in the onset and emergence of teenage attitudes and behavior regarding alcohol" (p. 167).

Programs must take advantage of peer pressure in a positive manner. To be nonjudgmental and to develop self-esteem in these vulnerable youths are goals of utmost importance and urgency. In program planning there is a need for youth to provide input regarding what they feel are their greatest stresses and programs needed to directly address these issues. Many youths use drugs as a coping mechanism. School pressures and adolescent growth (both emotional and physical) are all basic life problems. The schools can offer meaningful alternatives to drug use to help adolescents deal with these stressors. A variety of activities can be offered by schools to provide reinforcements for teenagers other than drugs. These after-school programs will be successful when they center on the youths' interests such as music, fashion, sports, and so forth. For example, gyms can be kept open on weekends and during summer months: a small price compared to the cost of consequences of drugs.

The problem in reaching these adolescents comes when they do not see their drug use as a problem but as a regular boredom-relieving activity. When drug-using youth are asked if they see their drug use as a problem, the most frequently encountered reply is "no" (Turanski, 1983). When they do recognize a problem, youth are ill-prepared to seek help. They are more often than not unaware of drug prevention and treatment centers. Moreover, they may view these services with mistrust, fear, and embarrassment. Another great fear is exposure to both parents and the law. Thus, communication has to occur regarding services that are available. Service providers have to reach out to the youths who are at risk.

HOME AND FAMILY

That "kids will learn what you tell them about drinking" is a myth that must be dispelled according to the United States Jaycees' Operation THRESHOLD pamphlet, "Drinking Myths." The fact is that "your kids will learn what you show them about drinking. If you drink heavily; if you get drunk; the chances are your kids will follow the same example." Thus, the mandate is clear that parents must set examples for their children. Young people need positive role models from which to gain their experiences. Data indicate that adolescents are more likely to consume drugs in a manner similar to that of their parents (Wodarski & Hoffman, 1984) and the parents' drug behavior is an important influence (Bacon & Jones, 1968).

The family is the "crucial influence on children's values and behavior." In the home, youth can find structure and guidance from loved ones who really care about them. Clear expectations about consumption can be communicated. Younger children are especially vulnerable to pressures and they need a trusting and comfortable place to turn for help in mastering their anxieties and frustrations. The home is the stabilizing influence for youth. It should be the place to turn where drug-induced states are not glorified.

Drinking is frequently associated with "coming of age" (Pittman & Snyder, 1962), and a driver's license and the availability of alcohol are symbols of adulthood. While forming their new identities, teens need "adult clarification and support in their process of becoming independent."

Parents must realize that in regard to drugs and driving they maintain ultimate control. Parents are the resource for the car availability. Mom and Dad have the power to keep the car away from abusing adolescents. Parents need to be reinforced regarding their responsibility and right to make decisions that are in the best interests of their children.

Parents may need help in asserting themselves and in coping with difficult situations. Support is available through such mechanisms as Parent Effectiveness Training (PET) classes where parents learn better parenting skills. Through such training, parents learn to set clear expectations about drugs and to enforce consequences when expectations are not met. Moreover, they practice ways to open lines of communication to discuss the use of drugs and their effects with their teenager.

MEDIA

The media exert a powerful influence on contemporary society. Examples of both positive and negative portrayals of substance abuse behavior in terms of setting appropriate expectations for drug consumption are aired throughout the viewing period. Depending on the programming, the messages are as varied as "drinking is mandated for a good time" and "to be a good friend, do not let your friend drink and drive." Young people "watch television and see the message of what they need and what they should want. 'Tuning in can lead to turning off by turning on'." Also, as Globetti (1977) suggests, "Adolescents . . . view drugs mostly in terms of sociability and in the sense of what it does for them rather than to them."

The significant impact of daytime and nighttime TV "soaps" needs to be evaluated. In these shows excessive consumption oftentimes is equated with power and success. In reality, adolescents must be informed that such consumption more likely impedes success. Many programs need parental interpretation.

The media can likewise exert a powerful positive influence. One of the favorite pastimes of contemporary youth is music. The messages this media conveys must be considered since it is a continual influence. Music can have a significant positive influence on youth. Positive role models affect the norms of youth and must be capitalized upon. Rather than glorify the consumption of drugs and its association with adventure and sex, role models can "turn on" teens to more positive outlets.

COMMUNITY MOVEMENTS

The ability to influence community norms rests within the community itself. By joining forces and establishing coalitions, standards of acceptance of substance abuse can be changed (Blansfield, 1984; Gardner, 1983).

Locally sponsored "Soberfests" have provided education and awareness about the impact of irresponsible drug use on society. In some communities, these events are sponsored by a coalition of "business, voluntary organizations, churches and synagogues, universities, tax-supported agencies, hospitals and medical facilities, civic organizations and others who have community wellness and a positive, aggressive, innovative approach to health" as a primary goal. They promote "new norms . . . stay alive; don't drink and drive; get high on life; and, it's OK not to drink" (Athens Community Wellness Council, 1984). Community-wide campaigns promote awareness of behaviors that "add enjoyment and years to life" and are a positive influence on community norms.

Other community organizations, such as the United States Jaycees with the Operation THRESHOLD, have taken steps to offer responsible alternatives to the norms that allow irresponsible drinking and driving under the influence. Mothers Against Drunk Drivers (MADD) is a grassroots organization that has succeeded in getting legislation passed for more adequate laws and enforcement. Such groups also provide social support necessary to sustain the work involved in these endeavors (Linblad, 1983).

LAWS AND ENFORCEMENT

Individual and community involvement and pressure can result in significant social change through governmental legislation and policy. On July 17, 1984, President Reagan signed into law a bill reducing federal highway aid to states that refused to raise the legal drinking age to 21 by the year 1986. This law also provides extra funding to states that penalize drunken drivers with automatic jail sentences and revoked licenses (*Atlanta Journal*, July 18, 1984). He changed his original stance on this issue after becoming aware that states that have raised their drinking age have seen a drop in alcohol-related accidents. Government officials, grassroots organizations, and private citizens provided the necessary push to get the legislation passed. With this new law came a clear, though long overdue, message to today's youth: drinking and driving is a problem that requires social action. Stronger enforcement of drug laws with absolute penalties is vital, with our government becoming more involved with source-country crop control and more taxation, interdiction efforts aimed at stopping illicit drugs at our border, and street-level enforcement through the use of physical surveillance or "buy and bust" operations (Saffer & Grossman, 1987; Moore, 1988).

BUSINESS AND INDUSTRY

Business and industry have shown concern about substance abuse. They have been spurred to action by data that indicate that productivity is substantially reduced when workers abuse substances (Mayer, 1983). Moreover, they are recognizing that work is a central aspect in many lives and that supportive business can foster positive attitudes concerning the consumption of substances. Their commitment has been expressed by repeated advertisements in the media. They are reaching a large number of markets through use of printed media, such as advertisements in major magazines. Business-sponsored radio and television spots also promote responsible drinking. These spots have been used especially during holiday periods when people of all ages celebrate by irresponsibly using alcohol.

CONCLUSION

The solution to the problem of substance abuse requires an all-out-effort by those societal forces capable of effecting change. Families, schools, peers, communities, businesses, and the media all possess powers to eradicate this social problem. The campaign cannot be waged from only one front, however. Combined cooperative efforts are essential. The responsibility must be shared for both previous condoning of actions that have perpetuated the problem and for working toward mutual goals and solutions.

The incidence of adolescent substance abuse and practice limitations have been reviewed. Variables that might be altered to prevent abuse among clients have been discussed. The chapter reviewed the following: effective treatment paradigms, school and peer environment, home and family, the media, community movements, laws and enforcement, and business and industry in terms of how they can be employed to prevent substance abuse. The chapter concluded with an elucidation of what must minimally be done to reduce adolescent substance abuse in America.

DICTIONARY OF COMMUNICATION TARGETS

Problematic Behavior	Possible Alternative
1. Talking through a third person.	Talking directly to another person.
2. Accusing, blaming, defensive statements.	Making I-statements (I feel _____ when _____ happens).
3. Putting down, zapping, shaming.	Accepting responsibility, I-statement.
4. Interrupting (other than for clarification).	Listening; raising hand or gesturing when wanting to talk. Encouraging speakers to use brief statements.
5. Overgeneralizing, catastrophizing, making extremist, rigid statements.	Qualifying, making tentative statements (sometimes, maybe, etc.); accurate quantitative statements.
6. Lecturing, preaching, moralizing.	Making brief, explicit problem statements (I would like _____).
7. Talking in a sarcastic tone of voice.	Talking in a neutral tone of voice.
8. Failing to make eye contact.	Looking at the person with whom you are talking.
9. Fidgeting, moving restlessly, or gesturing while being spoken to.	Sitting in a relaxed fashion. Excusing self for being restless.
10. Mindreading (attributing thoughts and feelings to another without the other's having communicated these feelings).	Reflecting, paraphrasing, validating.
11. Getting off the topic.	Catching self and returning to the problem as defined.
12. Commanding, ordering.	Suggesting alternative solutions.
13. Dwelling on the past.	Sticking to the present and future, suggesting changes to correct past problems.
14. Monopolizing the conversation.	Taking turns, making brief statements.

15. Intellectualizing, pedanticizing.	Speaking in simple, clear language that a teenager can understand.
16. Threatening.	Suggesting alternative solutions.
17. Humoring, discounting.	Reflecting, validating.
18. Incongruence between verbal and nonverbal behavior.	Matching verbal affect and nonverbal posture.

REFERENCES

Alcohol Health and Research World (March 3, 1983).

Adler, I. & Kandel, D.B. (1982). A cross-cultural comparison of sociopsychological factors in alcohol use among adolescents in Israel, France, and the United States. *Journal of Youth and Adolescence, 11*, 89-113.

Allen, T.J. (1983). The school as a family support system. *The U.S. Journal of Drug and Alcohol Dependence, 6*(3), 4.

Athens Community Wellness Council (1984). *Up with Wellness*, Athens, GA: Author.

Atlanta Journal (July 18, 1984).

Bacon, M. & Jones, M.B. (1968). *Teenage Drinking.* New York: Thomas Y. Crowell Company.

Bandura, A. (1969). *Principles of Behavior Modification*, New York: Holt, Rinehart & Winston.

Barr, H., Antes, D., Ottenberg, D., & Rosen, A. (1984). The morality of treated alcoholics and drug addicts: The benefits of sobriety. *Journal of Studies on Alcohol, 45*(5), 440-452.

Blansfield, H.N. (1984). Drinking and/or driving. *Connecticut Medicine, 48*(3), 205.

Botvin, G.J. (1983). Prevention of adolescent substance abuse through the development of personal and social competence. In *Preventing Drug Abuse: Intervention Strategies* [DHHS Publications No. (ADM) 83-1280]. Washington, DC: U.S. Government Printing Office.

Bronfenbrenner, U. (1974). The origins of alienation. *Scientific American, 231*, 53-61.

Dembo, R. & Burgos, W. (1976). A framework for developing drug abuse prevention strategies for young people in ghetto areas. *Journal of Drug Education, 6*(4), 313-325.

Elliott, D.S., Huizinga, D., & Menard, S. (1989). *Multiple Problem Youth Delinquency, Substance Use and Mental Health Problems.* New York: Springer-Verlag.

Fors, S.W. & Rojek, D.G. (1983). The social and demographic correlates of adolescent drug use patterns. *Journal of Drug Education, 13*, 205-222.

Gardner, S.E. (1983). *Communities: What You Can Do About Drug & Alcohol Abuse* (DHHS Pub. No. ADM 84-1310). Rockville, MD: National Institute on Drug Abuse.

Globetti, G. (1977). Teenage drinking. In N.J. Estes and M.E. Heinemann (Eds.), *Alcoholism: Development Consequences and Interventions.* St Louis: C.V. Mosby Company.

Hawkins, J.D., Abott, R., Catalano, R.F., & Gillmore, M.R. (1991). Assessing effectiveness of drug abuse prevention: Long-term effects and replication. In C. Leukefeld & W. Bukoski (Eds.), *Drug Abuse Prevention Research: Methodological Issues* (NIDA Research Monograph Series No. 107, DHHS Publication No. ADM 91-1761, pp. 195-212). Washington, DC: U.S. Government Printing Office.

Hawkins, J.D., Lishner, D.M., Jenson, J.M., & Catalano, R.F. (1987). Delinquents and drugs: What the evidence suggests about prevention and treatment programming. In B.S. Brown & A.R. Mills (Eds.), *Youth at High Risk for Substance Abuse* (DHHS Publication No. ADM 87-1537, pp. 81-133). Washington, DC: U.S. Government Printing Office.

Hill, J.P. (1980). The family. In M. Johnson (Ed.), *Toward Adolescence: The Middle School Years.* Chicago: University of Chicago Press.

Hirschi, T. (1969). *Causes of Delinquency.* Berkeley: University of California Press.

Janvier, R.L., Guthman, D.R., & Catalano, R.F. (1980). *An Assessment of Drug Abuse Prevention Programs,* Washington, DC: U.S. Superintendent of Documents, National Institute of Juvenile Justice and Delinquency Prevention.

Johnson, N. (1984). Research reports: Reducing community alcohol problems. *Alcohol Health and Research World, 8*(3), 60-61.

Kandel, D. (1974). Inter- and intra-generational influences on adolescent marijuana use. *Journal of Social Issues, 30,* 107-135.

Kandel, D. (1980). Developmental stages in drug involvement. In D. Lettieri (Ed.), *Theories of Drug Abuse* [NIDA Research Monograph Series, No. 30, DHHS Publication No. (ADM) 80-96]. Washington, DC: U.S. Government Printing Office.

Kandel, D., Kessler, R., & Margulies, R. (1978). Adolescent initiation into stages of drug use: A developmental analysis. In D. Kandel (Ed.) *Longitudinal Research on Drug Use: Empirical Findings on Methodological Issues.* Washington, DC: Hemisphere-Wiley.

Kandel, D., Simcha-Fagan, O., & Davies, M. (1986). Risk factors for delinquency and illicit drug use from adolescence to young adulthood. *The Journal of Drug Issues, 16,* 67-90.

Kane, R.L. & Patterson, E. (1972). Drinking attitudes and behavior of high school students in Kentucky. *Quarterly Journal of Studies on Alcohol, 33*(3), 635-646.

Kinder, B.N., Pape, N.E., & Walfish, S. (1980). Drug and alcohol education programs: A review of outcome studies. *The International Journal of the Addictions, 15*(7), 1035-1054.

Lewis, C.E. & Lewis, M. (1984). Peer pressure and risk taking behaviors in children. *American Journal of Public Health, 74*(6), 580-584.

Linblad, R.A. (1983). *Bulletin on Narcotics, 35*(3), 41-52.

Lowman, C., Hubbard, R.L., Rachel, J.V., & Cavanaugh, E.R. (1982). Facts for planning: Adolescent marijuana and alcohol use. *Alcohol Health and Research World, 6*(3), 69-75.

Mackay, J.R. (1961). Clinical observation on adolescent problem drinkers. *Quarterly Journal of Studies on Alcohol, 22,* 124-134.

Mayer, J.E. & Filstead, W.J. (1980). *Adolescence and Alcohol.* Cambridge, MA: Ballinger Publishing Co.

Mayer, W. (1983). Alcohol abuse and alcoholism: The psychologist's role in prevention, research, and treatment. *American Psychologist, 38*(10), 1116-1121.

Montemayor, R. (1982). The relationship between parent-adolescent conflict and the amount of time adolescents spend alone with parents and peers. *Child Development, 53,* 1512-1519.

Moore, M. (1988). *Drug Trafficking* (Crime File Study Guide), Washington, DC, U.S. Department of Justice, National Institute of Justice.

Morrison, M.A. (1985). Adolescence and vulnerability to chemical dependence. *Insight 1,* Atlanta, GA: Ridgeview Institute.

Morrison, M.A. & Smith, T.Q. (1987). Psychiatric issues of adolescent chemical dependence. *Pediatric Clinics of North America, 34*(2):461-480.

National Institute on Drug Abuse (1985). *National Household Survey on Drugs,* Washington, DC: Author.

Okel, S. (March 15, 1984). Number one killer of youth. *The Georgia Bulletin,* p. 11.

Patterns of Drug Use (1987-88 Fall/Winter). *ISR Newsletter,* p. 3, 6.

Pentz, M.A. (1983). Prevention of adolescent substance abuse through social skill development. In T. Glynn, C. Leukenfeld, & J. Ludford (Eds.), *Preventing Adolescent Drug Abuse: Intervention Strategies* (NIDA Research Monograph 47). Rockville, MD:DHHS.

Peterson, A.C. & Hamburgh, B.A. (1986). Adolescence: A developmental approach to problems and psychopathology. *Behavior Therapy, 17*(5), 480-499.

Pittman, D.J. & Snyder, C.R. (Eds.) (1962). *Society, Culture and Drinking Patterns.* Carbondale: Southern Illinois University Press.

Prendergast, T.J. & Schafer, E.F. (1974). Correlates of drinking and drunkenness among high school students. *Quarterly Journal of Studies on Alcohol, 35,* 232-242.

Robin, A.D. & Foster, S.L. (1989). *Negotiating Parent-adolescent Conflict: A Behavioral Family Systems Approach.* New York: Guilford Press.

Saffer, H. & Grossman, M. (1987). Beer taxes, the legal drinking age, and youth motor vehicle fatalities. *Journal of Legal Studies, 16,* 351-374.

Schinke, S. P., Bebel, M.Y., Orlandi, M.A., & Botvin, G.J. (1988). Prevention strategies for vulnerable pupils: School social work practices to prevent substance abuse. *Urban Education, 22,* 510-519.

Schinke, S.P. & Gilchrist, L.D. (1984). *Life Skills Counseling with Adolescents*, Baltimore: University Park Press.

Smith, K.A. & Forehand, R. (in press). Parent and adolescent conflict: Comparison and prediction of the perceptions of mothers, fathers, and daughters in a non-clinic sample. *Journal of Early Adolescence*.

Sutherland, E. & Cressey, D. (1970). *Criminology,* Philadelphia: J.B. Lippincott Company.

Swift, C.F. (1988). Stopping the violence: Prevention strategies for families. In L.A. Bond & B.M. Wagner (Eds.), *Families in Transition, Primary Prevention Programs that Work: Primary Prevention of Psychopathology,* (Vol. 11, pp. 252-285). Newbury Park, CA: Sage.

Swisher, J.D. (1976). An educational policy for school prevention: Rationale and research. *Contemporary Policy Issues, 4,* 27-35.

Turanski, J.J. (1983). Researching and treating youth with alcohol related problems: A comprehensive approach. *Alcohol Health and Research World, 7*(4), 3-9.

West, L.J., Maxwell, D.S., Noble, E.D., & Solomon, D.H. (1984). *Alcoholism Annals of Internal Medicine, 100*(3), 405-416.

Wodarksi, J.S. & Fisher, A.P. (1986). The alteration of adolescent DWI: A macro approach. *Alcoholism Treatment Quarterly, 3*(2), 153-162.

Wodarski, J.S. & Hoffman, S.D. (1984). Alcohol education for adolescents. *Social Work in Education, 6*(2), 69-2.

Chapter 2

Teams-Games-Tournaments Intervention

A unique adolescent education program, Teams-Games-Tournaments (TGT), has been developed for use by school professionals to teach adolescents about alcohol to prevent its misuse. TGT was developed through extensive research on games used as teaching devices, using small groups as classroom work units, and emphasizing the task-and-reward structures used in the traditional classroom. The TGT technique is an alternative teaching approach that fully utilizes a structure emphasizing group, rather than individual, achievement and utilizes peers as teachers and supporters of pro-social norms (Feldman & Wodarski, 1975; Wodarski, 1981; Wodarski et al., 1980). Thus, the TGT method capitalizes on peer influence, subsequently increases social attachment to peers which research suggests is a major influencing factor in an adolescent's life, and influences the acquisition and subsequent maintenance of knowledge and behavior change.

Results of a large-scale study by Wodarski (1987a, 1987b, 1988) support the effectiveness of TGT as a prevention strategy for alcohol abuse. In a study involving five school systems, high school students participated in a four-week educational program that focused on alcohol information and the application of the concepts to their own lives. The program emphasized behavioral objectives attained through self-management skills that lead to responsible drinking practices. Included in the study were three groups: students receiving the TGT method, those receiving traditional instruction, and those receiving no instruction. A total of 1,400 subjects participated. The results indicated that the TGT method was superior to the remaining groups in terms of each of the following self-report measures: alcohol knowledge, reduction in drinking behavior, positive changes concerning drinking and driving, reduced impulsivity, and improvement in several self-concept measures. In addition, both teacher and student evaluations indicated that the TGT program was viewed as a positive and productive experience. A one- and two-year follow-up indicates all of the effects of the TGT method on knowledge and attitudes were maintained (Wodarski, 1987b, 1987c). Based on these positive results and other data, it would appear that TGT programs could be used for drug, as well as for alcohol, prevention programs and is the most effective method for altering a peer support system which in many instances supports drug usage (Klepp, Halper, & Perry, 1986).

IMPLEMENTATION OF THE TGT
SUBSTANCE ABUSE PROGRAM

Adolescents participate in a six-week educational program focused on the understanding of drug information and the application of concepts to their own lives. The program emphasizes behavioral objectives aimed at acquisition of self-management skills. The completion of the assessment of drug knowledge provides the basis for dividing students into four-member teams. The teams are organized into high achievers (those with a high level of drug knowledge), middle achievers (those with moderate levels), and low achievers (those most lacking in drug knowledge). The composition of the teams is heterogeneous, including one high achiever, two middle achievers, and one low achiever. Thus, the average achievement level is approximately equal across teams. The achievement levels of individual students on the assessment of drug knowledge is not revealed.

The drug education units contained in the curriculum guide are presented for 50 minutes each day for six weeks. The first three days of each week are devoted to learning drug concepts by discussions and various participatory activities. The fourth day focuses on working in the TGT teams on worksheets, in preparation for the tournament to be held on the fifth day of each week.

The tournament games consist of short-answer questions designed to reinforce and assess the knowledge gained in class. These are played by team members individually competing against other team members of comparable achievement levels. The team members are assigned to a tournament table, competing against two students of comparable achievement levels from other teams. Scores are kept for each individual during the tournament games. At the end of the tournament, the top, middle, and low scorers at each table are awarded a fixed number of points for their teams. The points earned determine whether a student will stay at the same tournament table or move to a table with higher or lower performing students for the next tournament. In this way competitors change regularly, and the competition is not skewed in favor of any group of achievers. The points earned by an individual are added to those earned by other team members to compose a total team score. Teachers tabulate team scores at the end of each tournament, and scores are posted on the next school day.

The special timeliness of TGT to teach adolescents about alcohol and drugs and how to make better decisions regarding their usage is that when TGT is used, all students have an equal opportunity to succeed, because all students compete against members of other teams who are of similar achievement levels, and points earned by low achievers are just as valuable to the overall team score as points earned by high achievers. This is in contrast to the typical instructional method which centers on individual assessment compared to the total class. Thus, relative to individual instruction, the TGT method helps one of the high-risk populations for substance abuse (i.e., the low achieving student) to acquire knowledge. Moreover, there is significance in using the group reward structure with adolescents, in that it capitalizes on peer influence and reinforcement, which is considered to be one of the most potent variables in the acquisition, alteration, and maintenance of behavior in youth (Buckholdt & Wodarski, 1978).

The program of comprehensive drug education consists of the following components.

A. Drug Education

(1) Biological, psychological, and sociocultural determinants of drug abuse. It is crucial that in learning about drugs, participants become informed of the multiple factors that have been shown to contribute to irresponsible use of drugs and to dependence. This

will serve to assist participants in making realistic judgments about their own present or possible future drug use, and to inform them of the progression of drug use from responsible, to problem usage, to dependence. Adolescents have been found to lack such knowledge (Kaplan, Martin, & Robbins, 1984).

(2) Basic knowledge about drug consumption and usage. Students learn the gamut of topics related to drug use, such as the quantity of drugs a body can absorb in a given length of time, when an intoxicated person is in an emergency situation and how to deal with such an occurrence, the physiological attributes of drugs in relation to the human body, the amount of alcohol in a variety of alcoholic beverages, and how to assess a drug problem.

(3) Curriculum
    a. Drugs and Our Society
    b. What Are Drugs?
    c. Short-Term Effects of Drugs: Intoxication and Hangover
    d. Values Clarification and Drugs
    e. Common Motivations for Drugs and Drug Behavior
    f. Long-Term Effects of Drugs
    g. Drugs and the Effects on Driving
    h. Alternatives to Drugs in Our Society
    i. Recognizing and Treating Drug Problems

Both areas, determinants of drug abuse and basic knowledge, are taught via group discussion, participatory activities, and the TGT tournaments, all emphasizing the use of peer support to enhance learning and the acceptance of responsible attitudes toward drugs.

B. Self-Management and Maintenance

Students are taught basic principles of social learning theory related to drug consumption from a self-management of life perspective. Social learning theory oriented psychologists emphasize that the abuse of drugs is learned from the consequences that follow. These most often include: (1) stress reduction (the reinforcer might be lessened inhibition in sociability around peers); (2) removal from an unpleasant situation (given that adolescents tend to abuse more at one sitting than adults, this behavior more often results in their passing out to avoid dealing with an unpleasant situation); and (3) an excuse for otherwise unacceptable behavior (the person being un-usually aggressive or flirtatious could be excused on the basis of being intoxicated).

Other potential reinforcers for drug abuse are in abundance: modeling peer drug use in order to gain acceptance, peer pressure to drink or take drugs and subsequent reinforcement by significant peers, having fun equated with how much one drinks, and the need to escape from thought of academic failure.

A fundamental theme students learn is that one can change or determine behavior by altering one's environment and thus devel-oping different options for rewards. This may be the internal envi-ronment or the external environment. The two major categories of environmental events which must be understood and manipulated to produce the desired outcome are events which precede and set the stage for particular behaviors, and events which follow the behavior and make them more or less likely to occur (Williams & Long, 1979). Thus, one task of the learning experience of the pro-posed program is to help students identify environmental events controlling behavior and to alter the ones necessary to produce the desired behavior.

Examples of external environmental stimuli which cue substance abuse behaviors are parties or peer modeling of drug use. Examples of internal environmental events are emotional upset and loneliness. Students are instructed in how to remove or reduce stress-producing cues, such as irrational beliefs and faulty assessment of others' behavior from the environment and how to engage in rewarding activities other than the consumption of drugs (Botvin, Baker, Bot-vin, Filazzola, & Millman, 1984).

A necessary aspect of self-management particularly pertinent to drugs and their use is learning to be assertive with others (Horan & Williams, 1982). Recent research has shown that young adult prob-lem drug abusers often feel dissatisfaction with their interpersonal relationships with others and perceive themselves as lacking in social skills (Wodarski, 1993; Wodarski & Wodarski, 1993).

The adolescent learns how to better cope with the task of interact-ing with others in a meaningful and satisfying way. Facets of this program developed by Lange and Jakubowski (1976) are used. These involve conversational skills training, use of appropriate nonverbal communication, and development of assertive behavior in learning to decrease stress produced by inadequately met social needs.

Specific elements emphasized are how to: introduce oneself, initiate and continue conversations, give and receive compliments, enhance appearance, make and refuse requests, express feelings spontaneously, use appropriate nonverbal behavior in enhancing sociability with others, reward oneself for not drinking or taking drugs, and discuss alternatives for help with a significant other with a drinking or drug problem. Role-play simulation exercises are used to help adolescents practice how to refuse drugs in a socially acceptable manner within normal peer contexts. This aspect of the program is modeled after the work of Foy, Miller, Eisler, and O'Toole (1976). General procedures are referred to as drink/drug refusal training. The basic aim is to help students develop more effective ways of dealing with social pressures to consume drugs. Specific situations are practiced where individuals apply pressure to persuade others to consume excessive amounts of drugs. Students practice reactions to statements like: "One drink and/or pill won't hurt you." "What kind of friend are you?" or "Just have a little one; I'll make sure you won't have any more."

These areas of self-management skills are taught through group discussion and participatory activities and, where appropriate, are incorporated into the TGT tournaments.

Adolescents also need training in terms of coping with the daily problems of living: i.e., their academic and social concerns. They are taught a problem-solving approach based on the work of Robin and Foster (1984).

The general components emphasized are:

1. problem definition
2. how to generate possible solutions
3. decision making
4. how to choose and implement strategies through the following procedures:
   a. general introduction as to how the provision of certain consequences and stimuli can control problem-solving behavior

    b. isolation and definition of a behavior to be changed
    c. use of stimulus control techniques to influence rates of problem-solving behavior
    d. use of appropriate consequences to either increase or decrease a behavior
  5. verification of the outcome and renegotiation

Other essential components of the curriculum include stress management and relaxation training.

FAMILY PREVENTION STRATEGY

Parents participate in a five-week program in which they will meet in groups of ten families (both parents, if possible) two hours each week. Like the TGT procedures, the initial focus is on learning drug concepts. This information is dispensed in handouts and is discussed within the first two-hour group session. Topics covered include the amount of drugs the body can absorb in a given length of time, when an intoxicated person is in an emergency situation and how to deal with such an occurrence, the physiological attributes of drugs in relation to the human body, the amount of alcohol in various alcoholic beverages, and how to assess a drug problem. Also, long- and short-term effects of drugs and various types of drugs that are available are covered.

During the second session basic knowledge about drug consumption and usage is continued from the first session. Variables that initiate and maintain drug usage are covered. In addition, data on parental use of drugs and its effects on adolescents' drug use are elaborated.

The third and fourth sessions are devoted to teaching problem-solving skills and communication skills for conflict resolution (Robin & Foster, 1984). The five steps involved in problem solving are delineated: problem definition, generation of alternate solutions, decision making, planning solution implementation, and renegotiation. Based on Robin and Foster (1984) parents are initially presented with these steps in the following way. Ideas are presented in lecture form and then discussed in the group; next, teaching how to use the procedures through role playing is implemented. The role playing consists of selected group members attempting to solve problems of adolescents of other group members.

When the basic steps for problem solving have been delineated and practiced, communication training is implemented with particular emphasis on listening carefully, using reflective statements, reaching agreements before terminating a discussion, and using contracts. The communication targets (Robin & Foster, 1984) listed in Chapter 1 will be distributed to parents. The various problematic behaviors are discussed as well as the possible alternatives. Presentation of problematic and appropriate behavior is conducted by group leaders. Subsequently, various participants role play problem-solving situations and receive feedback from other group members concerning their use of communication/conflict resolution skills.

In sessions three and four, information is delineated on use of positive and negative control with adolescents. The focus within this material is on increasing use of positive reinforcement for appropriate behavior rather than often-used coercive processes such as negative reinforcement and punishment (Forehand & McMahon, 1981).

In the fifth session, the use of problem solving, communication training, and positive reinforcement procedures are integrated and applied to drug and alcohol prevention. It is emphasized to parents that generally using communication skills, problem-solving skills, and positive reinforcement will result in a better relationship with their adolescents (better communication, less conflict) and, therefore, reduce the probability of drug and alcohol use. However, it is also emphasized that these skills can be utilized directly in order to discuss drug and alcohol use and to implement solutions if drug and alcohol use is occurring.

SUMMARY

This chapter has elaborated the mechanics of Team, Games, and Tournaments. Method curriculum equip adolescents with necessary knowledge and relevant social skills to avoid and neutralize risk situations. The family component to support the education and skills aspects of the prevention intervention was reviewed.

REFERENCES

Botvin, G.H., Baker, E., Botvin, E.M., Filazzola, A.D., & Millman, R.B. (1984). Prevention of alcohol misuse through the development of personal and social competence: A pilot study. *Journal of Studies on Alcohol, 45*(6), 550-552.

Buckholdt, D. & Wodarski, J.S. (1978). The effects of different reinforcement systems on cooperative behavior exhibited by children in classroom contexts. *Journal of Research and Development in Education, 12*(1), 50-68.

Feldman, R.A. & Wodarski, J.S. (1975). *Contemporary Approaches to Group Treatment,* San Francisco: Jossey-Bass.

Forehand, R. & McMahon, R.J. (1981). *Helping the Non-compliant Child: A Clinician's Guide to Parent Training*, New York: Guilford.

Foy, C.W., Miller, P.M., Eisler, R.M., & O'Toole, O.H. (1976). Social skills training to teach adolescents to refuse drinks effectively. *Journal of Studies on Alcohol, 37* (9), 1340-1345.

Horan, J.J. & Williams, J.M. (1982). Longitudinal study of assertion training as a drug abuse prevention strategy. *American Educational Research Journal, 19*(3), 341-351.

Kaplan, H.B., Martin, S.S., & Robbins, C. (1984). Pathways to adolescent drug use: self-controls and early substance use. *Journal of Health and Social Behavior, 25*, 270-289.

Klepp, K., Halper, A., & Perry, C.L. (1986). The efficacy of peer leaders in drug abuse prevention. *Journal of School Health, 56*, 407-411.

Lange, A.J. & Jakubowski, P. (1976). *Responsible Assertive Behaviors.* Champaign, IL: Research Press.

Robin, A.D. & Foster, S.L. (1989). *Negotiating Parent-Adolescent Conflict: A Behavioral Family Systems Approach.* New York: Guilford Press.

Williams, R.L. & Long, J.D. (1979). *Toward a Self-Managed Lifestyle.* Boston Houghton Mifflin Co.

Wodarski, J.S. (1981). *Role of Research in Clinical Practice.* Baltimore: University Park Press.

Wodarski, J.S. (1987a). Teaching adolescents about alcohol and driving: A two-year follow up. *Journal of Drug Education, 17*(4), 327-344.

Wodarski, J.S. (1987b). A social learning approach to teaching adolescents about drinking and driving: A multiple variable follow-up evaluation. *Journal of Behavior Therapy and Experimental Psychiatry, 18*(1), 51-60.

Wodarski, J.S. (1992-93). Teaching adolescents about alcohol and driving: An empirically validated program for social workers. *Research on Social Work Practice, 4*(1), 28-39.

Wodarski, L.A., Adelson, C., Tidball, M., & Wodarski, J.S. (1980). Teaching nutrition by teams-games-tournaments. *Journal of Nutrition Education, 12*(2), 61-65.

Wodarski, J.S. & Wodarski, L.A. (1993). *Curriculums and Practical Aspects of Implementation: Preventive Health Services for Adolescents.* Lanham, MD: University Press of America.

Chapter 3

Adolescent Component of Prevention: The Intervention

Youth are making decisions about the role alcohol and drugs will play in their lives. This is a timely, large-looming decision every adolescent must face; hence, there is a crucial need for teenagers to have an accurate, broad, well-rounded foundation of knowledge to draw upon when making decisions about alcohol and drug use (Ramey, Bryant, Campbell, Sparling, & Wasik, 1988).

Most often, the contact point of visibility of adolescents facing alcohol and drug issues is the school setting where adolescents spend approximately 50 percent of their waking hours. School comprises the society of youth–in this arena parents are excluded; the rulers are peers, with teachers at best playing the role of consultants. The greater amount of quality time teachers and administrators devote to substance abuse education to assist adolescents in learning self-management skills related to substance use, the greater the likelihood of ensuring against a haphazard, hit-or-miss approach to adolescents' life decisions pertaining to substance use and abuse (Botvin & Wills, 1985; Kandel, 1986; Ladd & Asher, 1985).

Effective comprehensive methods of teaching youth about psychoactive substances are imperative if they are to make well-informed decisions about its use (Ellickson & Bell, 1990). In order to fully impact on youth, the most critical point for receptivity seems to be the early adolescent years–following the influence of the parental/home setting and coinciding with the influx of peer influence. If the peer group is met successfully with a sociocultural approach to change the social norms surrounding substance use, then peers can make knowledgeable, unpressured, individual decisions regarding the use of psychoactive substances.

The Comprehensive Psychoactive Substance Use Education Program for Adolescents is targeted to provide essential knowledge to adolescents about psychoactive substances in such a manner as to be a fun, peer group experience, thus increasing the likelihood of acquisition of knowledge and behavior. The program is comprised of three parts: education about psychoactive substances, self-management skills related to substance use, and the maintenance of knowledge and behavior. The instructional method of the comprehensive program is the Teams-Games-Tournaments (TGT) technique.

Before beginning the education phase of the program, students are assessed for level of psychoactive substance knowledge. The completion of the pretest of psychoactive substance knowledge (see Pretest pg. 34) will provide the basis for division of students into four-member teams. The teams will be organized into high achievers (those with a high level of psychoactive substance knowledge), middle achievers (those with moderate levels), and low achievers (those most lacking in psychoactive substance knowledge). Team composition will be heterogeneous, with one high achiever, two middle achievers, and one low achiever on each team, so that the average achievement level will be approximately equal across teams.

Behavioral analysis over the last 20 years has been applied to the solution of many classroom problems, including discipline and the teaching of verbal reading and arithmetic skills. This is the first curriculum study to teach substance abuse education to secondary students through behavioral analysis. TGT is preferred over individual classroom instruction substance abuse education for several reasons. First, the group-learning situation most closely resembles the setting in which adolescents make their decisions regarding the use of substances among peers. And since substance abuse most often takes place in group settings, knowledge acquired in the group setting is more likely to be used when in similar peer group settings than knowledge acquired through individual, separate means (Allman, Taylor, & Nathan, 1972; Botvin, Baker, Filazzola, & Botvin, 1990). From the perspective of the educator, the group method allows for a broader range of learning experience; students have the opportunity to learn while interacting with peers in a friendly, exciting game. Refer to Chapter 2 for a comprehensive discussion of the TGT method.

The psychoactive substance use education units provided in this guide are to be presented for 50 minutes each day for six weeks. The first three days of each week are to be devoted to learning the psychoactive substance concepts in the exercises, discussions, and various participatory activities. The fourth day is to be focused on working in the TGT teams on worksheets in preparation for the tournament which is to be held on the fifth day of each week.

PRETEST

1. Alcohol is:
   A. a stimulant
   B. an anesthetic
   C. a narcotic
   D. a sedative-hypnotic drug

2. The effects of stimulant abuse can cause:
   A. aggressive behavior
   B. panic
   C. hallucinations
   D. all of the above

3. The _____ metabolizes psychoactive substance.
   A. stomach
   B. liver
   C. kidneys
   D. gall bladder

4. The number of deaths annually that are directly attributable to substance abuse is:
   A. 15,000 to 20,000
   B. 8,000 to 10,000
   C. 100,000 to 120,000
   D. 45,000 to 50,000

5. Cocaine is:
   A. a hallucinogen
   B. a depressant
   C. a narcotic
   D. a stimulant

6. Which of the following is not accepted as a possible cause of chemical dependence?
   A. nutritional deficiency
   B. personality factors
   C. genetic deficiency
   D. a learned behavior

7. Heroin is synthesized from morphine and is _____ times as potent.
   A. 3   B. 10   C. 18   D. 35

8. In the later stages of chemical dependence, the person often has all but which characteristic?
   A. a system of alibis about why he/she drinks or uses
   B. an accepted belief that no one cares about him/her
   C. a lack of faith in religion
   D. a loss of self-respect

9. The two most commonly used and abused drugs in America are:
   A. alcohol and cocaine
   B. marijuana and depressants
   C. alcohol and heroin
   D. alcohol and marijuana

10. Teenagers use drugs:
    A. to have a good time
    B. to be part of the group
    C. to get their minds off of problems or escape
    D. all of the above

11. _____ is the most common contaminant found in a number of street drugs.
    A. PCP   B. codeine   C. heroin   D. crack

12. Two-thirds of high school students use alcohol and drugs with regular frequency. Of these, _____ percent use drugs and alcohol at least three times weekly.
    A. 15 percent   B. 85 percent   C. 33 percent   D. 50 percent

13. _____ is the only cure for intoxication.
    A. coffee   B. time   C. cold shower   D. carbonated drink

14. Research shows that motor skills and reaction time are reduced by _____ percent after smoking one marijuana cigarette.
    A. 5 percent   B. 17 percent   C. 41 percent   D. 25 percent

15. A form of amnesia, lasting from seconds to days, resulting from alcohol use is a:
    A. blackout   B. seizure   C. convulsion   D. delirium

16. _____ percent of all teen suicide attempts are via drug overdose.
    A. 15 percent   B. 73 percent   C. 29 percent   D. 88 percent

True or False:

17. A user becomes tolerant to chemicals and requires more and more to get the same high.
18. A slang term for amphetamines is uppers.
19. Sniffing inhalants can lead to sudden death.
20. Only the use of narcotics leads to drug addiction.

21. Withdrawal from alcohol or other depressants can result in death.
22. Cough syrups containing codeine are classified as depressants.
23. Marijuana use has been proven to result in cellular damage to the body.
24. Depressants used in combination with alcohol are not potentially fatal.
25. The repeated use of narcotics results in increased tolerance.
26. Moderate to heavy marijuana use by males results in a decreased sperm count and an abundance of abnormally formed sperm.
27. It is okay to take medication prescribed for someone else if you have similar symptoms.
28. Marijuana can be addicting.
29. People sometimes use psychoactive substances to feel part of a group.
30. When a person becomes high and drives, it is human nature that the person will become more cautious than normal.
31. If a chemically dependent person really wanted to, he/she could stop drinking or using to excess.
32. Society is very unified about the cause of psychoactive substance abuse/dependence.
33. Most chemically dependent people are men.
34. Withdrawal from narcotics produces physical discomfort but does not result in death.
35. An overdose of cannabis marijuana can produce psychosis.
36. The media does not really influence how people view using psychoactive substances.
37. Psychoactive substances get to the bloodstream almost as soon as they are ingested.
38. More teenagers die in drug- and alcohol-related motor vehicle accidents than from any disease.
39. Physical dependency means that a person would get withdrawal symptoms upon decreasing or ceasing the use of chemical substance.
40. A person cannot become addicted to prescription drugs.
41. Once psychoactive substances enter the brain they do not circulate back through the body again.
42. Studies have shown that chronic exposure to some solvents and gasoline causes severe anemia and leukemia.

43. The effects of marijuana on female reproduction are of short duration.
44. The intravenous injection of narcotics or other substances can result in hepatitis, AIDS, or other infections from contaminated needles.
45. Two reasons why people sometimes try to persuade friends to use drugs are to see the effects on someone else or because they do not want to use alone.
46. Heavy drinking for a long period of time may cause physical problems but does not cause brain damage.
47. Dependency on crack can occur in as little as two weeks.
48. When psychoactive substances are snorted or inhaled they go directly to the brain.
49. A strong cup of coffee will sober a person up after they have become high from using psychoactive substances.
50. When using stimulants, drivers tend to overreact at the wheel.
51. It is important for family members with a chemically dependent person in the family to talk to someone about how chemical dependency has affected their life.
52. Seventy percent of marijuana users drive while high.
53. LSD is a stimulant.
54. The effects of PCP can last up to days.

PRETEST ANSWER SHEET

1. D	13. B	25. True	37. True	49. False
2. D	14. C	26. True	38. True	50. True
3. B	15. A	27. False	39. True	51. True
4. C	16. D	28. True	40. False	52. True
5. D	17. True	29. True	41. False	53. False
6. A	18. True	30. False	42. True	54. True
7. B	19. True	31. False	43. False	
8. C	20. False	32. False	44. True	
9. D	21. True	33. False	45. True	
10. D	22. False	34. True	46. False	
11. A	23. True	35. True	47. True	
12. B	24. False	36. False	48. False	

WEEK I
DAY 1
ACTIVITY 1: DEFINING THE PROBLEM: PSYCHOACTIVE SUBSTANCE USE

Focus: Increase understanding of psychoactive substance
Method: Mini-lecture/discussion
Time: 1 period
Capsule Description: This exercise is designed to acquaint students with the concept of psychoactive drugs and to stimulate a discussion of various types of psychoactive substances.

1. A mini-lecture will be presented to the class to define the concept of psychoactive substances. Psychoactive substances are any chemical substances, including alcohol, which when ingested have an effect on thoughts, feelings, or behavior.

2. Have your students divide up into small groups and brainstorm their own lists of psychoactive drugs.

3. Following the small group brainstorming, the class as a whole can then develop a single master list incorporating all psychoactive substances identified.

4. Finally, have your students brainstorm at least one possible effect of each drug listed.

WEEK I
DAY 2
ACTIVITY 2: MAJOR CLASSIFICATIONS OF SUBSTANCES ABUSED

Focus: Develop understanding of the major classifications of psychoactive substances
Method: Developing a chart/discussion
Time: 1 period
Capsule Description: This exercise is designed to increase students' knowledge of commonly abused substances. Students will develop a substance abuse chart.

1. Have the class divided into six small groups. Group 1 will be narcotics, group 2–depressants, group 3–stimulants, group 4–hallucinogens, group 5–cannabis, and group 6–organic solvents.

2. Distribute to all group members blank copies of the Slang Terms and Symptoms of Abuse Chart. Also distribute to each group the information sheet (photocopied) pertinent to their topic. For example, the narcotics group will receive the narcotics information sheet, etc.

3. Have each small group discuss the information sheet and fill in that portion of the blank chart (ex: narcotics information form narcotics sheet).

4. Reconvene the class and have each small group present their topic to the rest of the class. Class members can fill in their blank charts as information is presented.

5. Close the session by allowing time for class discussion of the activity.

SLANG TERMS AND SYMPTOMS OF ABUSE CHART

Drug	Trade Names	Other Names	Medical Uses	Duration of Effects (in hours)	Usual Methods of Administration	Possible Effects	Effects of Overdose	Withdrawal Symptoms
Opium	Dovers Powder, Paregoric, Parepectolin	Opium	Analgesic, Antidiarrheal	3-6 hrs.	O, SM	Euphoria, Drowsiness, Respiratory Depression, Constricted Pupils, Nausea	Slow and Shallow Breathing, Clammy Skin, Convulsions, Coma, Possible Death	Watery Eyes, Runny Nose, Yawning, Loss of Appetite, Irritability, Tremors, Panic, Chills and Sweating, Cramps, Nausea
Morphine	Morphine Pectoral Syrup	M, Morpho, Morph, Tab, White Stuff, Miss Emma Monkey	Analgesic Antitussive		O, I, SM			
Codeine	Codeine, Empirin Compound with Codeine Robitussin A-C	School Boy	Analgesic Antitussive		O, I			
Heroin	Diacetylmorphine	Horse, Smack, H, Stuff, Junk	Under Investigation		I, SN, SM			
Hydromorphone	Dilaudid	Little D, Lords	Analgesic		O, I			
Meperidine (Pethidine)	Demerol Pethadol	Isonipecaine, Dolantin	Analgesic					
Methadone	Dolophine Methadone, Methadose	Dollies, Dolls, Amidone	Analgesic Heroin substitute	12-24 hrs.				

NARCOTICS

Category	Drug Names	Trade or Other Names	Medical Uses	Duration (hrs.)	Usual Method	Possible Effects	Effects of Overdose	Withdrawal Syndrome
Other Narcotics	Laam, Leritine, Levodromoran, Percodan, Tussionex, Fentanyl, Darvon, Talwin, Lomotil	T. and Blue's designer drugs (fentanyl derivatives) China White	Analgesic, Antidiarrheal, Antitussive	Variable	Oral Injected	Slurred speech, Disorientation Drunken Behavior without Odor of Alcohol	Shallow Respiration, Cold and Clammy Skin, Dilated Pupils, Weak and Rapid Pulse, Coma	Anxiety, Insomnia, Tremors Delirium, Convulsions, Possible Death
Barbiturates	Amobarbital, Phenobarbital, Butisol, Secobarbital, Tuinal	Yellows, Yellow Jackets, Barbs, Reds, Redbirds, Tooies, Phennies	Anesthetic, Anti-convulsant Sedative, Hypnotic	1-16 hrs.				
Methaqualone		Lune, Quay, Quad, Mandrex	None (production discontinued in 1984)	4-8 hrs.				
Benzo-diazepines	Activan, Azene, Clonopin, Dalmane, Diazepam, Librium, Serax, Tranxene, Valium, Verstran	Downers, Goof Balls, Sleeping pills, Candy	Anti-Anxiety, Anti-convulsant, Sedative, Hypnotic					
Other Depressants	Equanil, Miltown Noludar, Placidylvalmid	Tranquilizers, muscle relaxants, sleeping pills	Anti-Anxiety, Sedative, Hypnotic					

DEPRESSANTS

Drug	Trade Names	Other Names	Medical Uses	Duration of Effects (in hours)	Usual Methods of Administration	Possible Effects	Effects of Overdose	Withdrawal Symptoms
STIMULANTS								
Cocaine	Cocaine	Bump, Toot, C, Coke, Flake, Snow, Candy	Local anesthetic	1-2 hrs.	O, I, SM, SN	Increased Alertness, Excitation, Euphoria, Increased Pulse Rate and Blood Pressure, Insomnia, Loss of Appetite	Agitation, Increase in body Temperature, Hallucinations, Convulsions, Possible Death	Apathy, Long Period of Sleep, Irritability, Depression, Disorientation
Amphetamines	Bithetamine, Delobese, Desoxyn, Dexeprine, Mediatric	Pep Pills, Bennies, Uppers, Truck Drivers, Dexies, Black Beauties, Speed	Hyperkinesis, Narcolepsy, Weight Control	2-4 hrs.	Oral Injected			
Phemmetrazine	Preludin	Uppers, Peaches, Hearts						
Metham-phetamine		Speed, Meth, Crystal, Crank, Go Fast						
HALLUCINOGENS								
LSD	Lysergic Acid Diethylamide	Acid, Microdot, Cubes	None	8-12 hrs.	Oral	Illusions and Hallucinations, Poor Perception of Time and Distance	Longer More Intense Trip Episodes, Psychosis, Possible Death	Withdrawal Syndrome not Reported
Mescaline and Peyote		Mesc, Buttons, Cactus			Oral, Injected			
Amphetamine Variants	2,5-DMA, PMA, STP, MDA, MDMA, TMA, DOM, DOB	Ecstasy, Designer Drugs						
Phencyclidine	Phencyclidine	PCP, Angel Dust, Hog, Peace, Pill	Veterinary Anesthetic	Up to Days	Oral, Injected			

	Drug			Medical Use	Duration	Administration	Possible Effects	Effects of Overdose	Withdrawal Syndrome
	Other Hallucinogens	DMT, DET, Psilocybin, Psilocyn	Sacred Mushrooms, Magic Mushrooms	None	Variable	O, I, SM, SN			
CANNABIS	Marijuana	Acapulco Gold, Sinsemilla, Thai Sticks	Pot, Grass, Reefer, Roach Maui Wowie, Joint, Weed, Loco Weed, Mary Jane	Under Investigation	2-4 hrs.	Smoked, Oral	Euphoria, Relaxed Inhibitions, Increased Appetite, Disoriented	Fatigue, Paranoia, Possible Psychosis	Insomia, Hyperactivity and Decreased Appetite, Occasionally Reported
CANNABIS	Tetrahydro-cannabinol	THC	THC						
CANNABIS	Hashish	Hash	Hash	None					
CANNABIS	Hashish Oil	Hash Oil	Hash Oil	None					
ORGANIC SOLVENTS	Inhalants	Gasoline, Airplane Glue, Veg. Spray, Hairspray, Deodorants, spray paint, Liquid paper Paint Thinner rubber cement	Sniffing, Glue Sniffing	None	30 min.	Sniffed	Euphoria, Headaches, Nausea, Fainting, Stupor, Rapid Heartbeat	Damage to Lungs, Liver, Kidneys, Bone Marrow, Suffocation, Choking, Anemia, Possible Stroke, Sudden Death	Insomia, Increased Appetite, Depression, Irritability, Headache

O=Oral, I=Injected, SM=Smoked, SN=Sniffed
Source: Curriculum and Practice Aspects of Implementation, John S. Wodarski and Lois Ann Wodarski.

SLANG TERMS AND SYMPTOMS OF ABUSE CHART

Drug	Trade Names	Other Names	Medical Uses	Duration of Effects (in hours)	Usual Methods of Adminis-tration	Possible Effects	Effects of Overdose	Withdrawal Symptoms
NARCOTICS								

DEPRESSANTS

DEPRESSANTS

Drug	Trade Names	Other Names	Medical Uses	Duration of Effects (In hours)	Usual Methods of Adminis-tration	Possible Effects	Effects of Overdose	Withdrawal Symptoms
STIMULANTS								
HALLUCINOGENS								

CANNABIS

ORGANIC SOLVENTS

47

WEEK I
DAY 3
ACTIVITY 3: SUBSTANCE ABUSE TERMS

Focus: Defining Abuse and Addiction
Method: Mini-lecture/role play
Time: 1 period
Capsule Description: This exercise is designed to enhance students' knowledge of substance abuse terminology. A mini-lecture followed by student role playing will be utilized.

1. Present to the class the substance abuse terms defined below.

2. After the presentation of the concepts, have the students divided into small groups and role play an example using each concept.

3. At the end of role play, reconvene the class and have students discuss the role play experience.

Terms and Definitions

1. *Drug dependence*–the state produced by repeated administration of a drug such that the drug user will engage in repeatable behavior patterns over an extended period of time with such behavior leading to further administration of the drug.

2. *Polydrug abuse*–the simultaneous or sequential use of more than one psychoactive drug for nonmedicinal purposes.

3. *Drug abuse*–the use of a drug, including alcohol, in a manner that deviates from the approved medical or social patterns within a given culture.

4. *Physical dependence*–an altered physiological state produced by the repeated administration of a drug, including alcohol, which necessitates the continued administration to prevent the appearance of withdrawal symptoms.

5. *Psychological dependence*–continued, repetitive use of the drug is required to maintain emotional or psychological equilibrium.

6. *Drug addiction*–a behavioral pattern of drug use characterized by overwhelming involvement with the use of a drug, compulsiveness in the securing of its supply, and a high tendency to relapse after withdrawal.

7. *Withdrawal symptom*–any of the symptoms caused by the with-

drawal of a physically addictive drug, such as tremors, sweating, chills, vomiting, seizures, and coma. Psychologically addictive drugs that, when withdrawn, can produce symptoms such as deep depression, anxiety, sense of helplessness, and an inability to function.

8. *Tolerance*–the state that develops when, after repeated administration, a given dose of a drug produces decreased effect or, conversely, when increasingly larger doses must be administered to obtain the effects observed with the original dose.

9. *Chemical Dependence*–a psychosocial, biogenetic disease–a chronic, progressive, familial, and relapsing disease that is fatal if untreated.

WEEK I
DAY 4
TEAM PRACTICE SESSION

Focus: Preparation for TGT tournament
Method: Worksheets
Time: 1 period
Capsule Description: The students work in their TGT teams on specially prepared worksheets in preparation for the TGT tournament.

Divide the class members into their TGT teams and let them work the worksheets in their small groups. Instruct the groups to discuss each question, coming to a consensus answer for each question. Circulate throughout the class to check the groups' progress and answer any questions. When all groups are finished with the worksheets, go over them as a class and provide them with correct answers so that they may study for the tournament tomorrow.

TEAM WORKSHEET I

1. True or False: Alcohol is a stimulant.

2. Name three types of psychoactive drugs.

3. True or False: A user becomes tolerant to chemicals and requires more and more to get the same high.

4. A slang term for amphetamines is _____ .

5. Name one possible effect of hallucinogen use.

6. Psychoactive drugs, when ingested, have an effect on thoughts, feelings, or _____ .

7. Weed and reefer are slang terms for what classification of drugs?

8. True or False: Sniffing of inhalants can lead to sudden death.

9. Name three methods for use of cocaine.

10. The continued or repetitive use of a drug in order to maintain psychological or emotional equilibrium is _____ .

11. True or False: Only the use of narcotics leads to drug addiction.

12. The effects of PCP can last how long?

13. Name two symptoms of an overdose of depressants.

14. True or False: Withdrawal from alcohol or other depressants can result in death.

15. Does marijuana have any known medical uses?

16. Name three effects of the use of stimulants.

17. True or False: Cough syrup containing codeine would be classified as a narcotic drug.

18. True or False: Withdrawal from narcotics produces physical discomfort but does not result in death.

19. The simultaneous use of more than one psychoactive drug for nonmedicinal purposes is called _____ .

20. True or False: An overdose of cannabis can produce psychosis.

ANSWERS TO TEAM WORKSHEET I

1. False
2. Alcohol, valium, speed, demerol, PCP, marijuana, cocaine, inhalants, etc.
3. True
4. Speed, Bennies, Uppers, Dexies, Black Beauties, Pep Pills, Truck Drivers
5. Illusion, hallucination, poor perceptions of time and distance
6. Behavior
7. Cannabis
8. True
9. Inhalation, smoking, injection, oral
10. Psychological dependence
11. False
12. Up to days
13. Shallow respiration, cold/clammy skin, dilated pupils, weak and rapid pulse, coma, possible death
14. True
15. Under investigation
16. Increased alertness, excitation, euphoria, increased pulse rate and blood pressure, insomnia, loss of appetite
17. True
18. True
19. Polydrug abuse
20. True

WEEK I
DAY 5
TOURNAMENT

Focus: Summarizing, integrating week's activities
Method: Game
Time: 1 period
Capsule Description: Students in their TGT teams compete for points by correctly answering questions based on the week's activities.

Divide the class into the tournament tables. Start the tournament by explaining the rules of play. Pass out copies of the "GIGS" to each team from the following page of this guide. When the students understand the game rules and instructions, pass out Game A, Game A Answer Sheet, and Game Score Sheet to each team. Answer any questions. At the end of the tournament, fill out the Team Summary Sheet and publicize the results. Then devise new tournament tables according to the "bumping" procedure.

GIGS: GENERAL INSTRUCTIONAL GAME STRUCTURE

MATERIAL NEEDED: (1) deck of question cards (to be made from list of questions on next page); (2) rules; (3) answer sheet

The Rules

1. To start the game, shuffle the deck of cards and place it face down on the table. Decide who will be player number 1. Play is clockwise from player number 1.
2. Each player (when it is his or her turn) must take the top card from the deck, read it aloud, and do one of two things:
   a. Answer the question immediately and ask if anyone wants to challenge the answer. The player to the right of the person giving the answer has the first chance to challenge. If he or she does not wish to challenge, the next player to the right can challenge.
   b. If he or she does not know the answer or is unsure of the answer, ask if another player wants to give an answer. If no one wants to give an answer, the card is placed on the bottom of the deck. If another player gives an answer, the procedure described above is followed.
3. If there is no challenge, another player should check the answer. In the lower right hand corner of each card, there is a letter and a number; use this to find the answer on the answer sheet.
   a. If the answer is correct, the player keeps the card.
   b. If the answer is wrong, the player must place the card on the bottom of the deck.

4. If there is a challenge and the challenger decides not to give an answer:
   a. If the original answer is wrong, the player must place the card on the bottom of the deck.
   b. If the original answer is correct, the player keeps the card and the challenger must give up one of the cards he or she has already won (if any) and place it on the bottom of the deck.
5. If there is a challenge and the challenger gives an answer:
   a. If the challenger's answer is correct, the challenger receives the card.
   b. If the challenger gives the wrong answer, and the original answer is correct, the challenger must give up one of the cards he or she has already won (if any) and place it on the bottom of the deck.
   c. If both the challenger's answer and the original answer are wrong, the card is placed on the bottom of the deck.
6. At the end of the game, when there are no more cards in the deck, each player counts up the number of cards he or she has and records this number as his or her score. The player who has the most cards is the winner.

GAME A
DEFINING THE PROBLEM:
PSYCHOACTIVE SUBSTANCE USE

A-1 True or False: Alcohol is a stimulant.

A-2 Name one possible effect of narcotic use.

A-3 Speed is a slang term for _____ .

A-4 True or False: Tolerance has developed when less use of the chemical involved results in the person getting high.

A-5 Name one possible effect of hallucinogen use.

A-6 Weed and reefer are slang terms for what classification of drugs?

A-7   Name two categories of psychoactive drugs.

A-8   True or False: An overdose of cannabis can result in psychosis.

A-9   The effects of PCP can last how long?

A-10 The effects of marijuana use for medicinal purposes is under investigation.

A-11 True or False: A strong pulse and increased alertness are symptoms of an overdose of depressants.

A-12 What is the most serious consequence of sniffing organic solvents?

A-13 Psychoactive drugs, when ingested, have an effect on thoughts, feelings, or _____ .

A-14 True or False: The simultaneous use of more than one psychoactive drug for nonmedicinal purposes is called polydrug abuse.

A-15 True or False: Only the use of narcotics leads to drug addiction.

A-16 Name three methods of cocaine use.

A-17 True or False: The continued or repetitive use of a drug in order to maintain psychological or emotional equilibrium is called psychological dependence.

A-18 Withdrawal from alcohol or other depressants can result in _____ .

A-19 True or False: Organic solvents have proven medicinal uses.

A-20 Can withdrawal from narcotics result in death?

A-21 What drug classification includes cough syrup with codeine?

A-22 True or False: All classifications of drugs, except hallucinogens, have reported withdrawal symptoms.

A-23 What are the six major classifications of psychoactive drugs?

GAME A ANSWER SHEET
DEFINING THE PROBLEM:
PSYCHOACTIVE SUBSTANCE USE

A-1 False
A-2 Euphoria, drowsiness, respiratory depression, constricted pupils, nausea
A-3 Amphetamines
A-4 False
A-5 Illusions, hallucinations, poor perception of time and distance
A-6 Cannabis
A-7 Narcotics, depressants, stimulants, hallucinogens, cannabis, organic solvents
A-8 True
A-9 For days
A-10 True
A-11 False
A-12 Sudden death
A-13 Behavior
A-14 True
A-15 False
A-16 Snorting, smoking, oral, injection
A-17 True
A-18 Death
A-19 False
A-20 No
A-21 Narcotics
A-22 True
A-23 Narcotics, depressants, stimulants, hallucinogens, cannabis, organic solvents

GAME SCORE SHEET

Date _____   Class _____

Tournament Table Number _____   Tournament Number _____

Names	Team	Day's Points	Tournament Pts.	Next Table
1.				
2.				
3.				
4.				
5.				

Absent Students:

1.

2.

TEAM SUMMARY SHEET

TEAM NAME _____

Pts. rec'd this tournament / Total rec'd to date

Team Members	Tournament Points						FINAL POINTS
	Date						
1.							
2.							
3.							
4.							
5.							
6.							
TOTALS							

WEEK II
EXPLORING PSYCHOACTIVE SUBSTANCE USE
DAY 1
ACTIVITY 4:
EXPLORING MARIJUANA, COCAINE, ALCOHOL USE

Focus: Physical, psychological effects of marijuana, cocaine, alcohol

Method: Role play/discussion

Time: 1 period

Capsule Description: This exercise is designed for role play in which the students review the substance abuse chart and role play the effects of the uses of these substances.

1. Divide the class into three groups: marijuana group, cocaine group, and alcohol group. Ask each group to review the substance abuse chart with particular attention to the substances used in their role play.

2. When small groups have finished, have each group present to the class a role play to provide information about the effects and consequences of the use of their particular substance. At the end of each role play have that group list on the blackboard behaviors and problems associated with the drug presented.

3. Following the role play of all three groups, have the entire class discuss their reactions to the role play and list any additional information regarding behaviors and problems associated with the use of each substance presented.

4. Present to the class a photocopied handout on marijuana, cocaine, and alcohol.

MARIJUANA

MARIJUANA is the term used in this country to refer to the *Cannabis Satavia L.* plant and to any part or extract of it. This plant grows wild in many temperate and tropical regions of the world, such as Mexico, the Middle East, Africa, and India. Due to its increasing value in the illegal drug market, marijuana is being grown in large quantities using modern agricultural techniques in areas where legal detection is difficult or lax.

The plant is a series of leaves that have odd numbered sets of leaflets (five, seven, nine, etc.). Marijuana can grow as tall as 20 feet in height. Even though marijuana has been known to man for thousands of years, its active ingredient, tetrahydrocannabinol (THC), was not synthesized until 1966.

SLANG TERMS. Pot, grass, weed, ganga, reefer, lid, smoke, joint, roach, Mary Jane, Loco Weed.

The unseen danger of marijuana is the possibility of substances such as PCP, heroin, or cocaine being sprayed on the leaves to enhance the marijuana high or obtain another type of high. This represents untold effects and dangers.

METHODS OF ABUSE. Marijuana is smoked in a variety of ways. Sometimes the user will roll the tobacco, like a cigarette, by hand. Sometimes the substance is smoked in a pipe, handmade or purchased. Many intricate pipes are now manufactured for this use. Users add marijuana to food substances such as brownies, or they may brew marijuana like tea. Hashish usually is smoked in a pipe.

EFFECTS. Marijuana ingestion produces various effects in different people and the high tends to last from two to four hours. Some people experience a light-headed, giddy feeling while others report depression and sadness. The user experiences distortion of time and depth perception. Behavior may become reckless or erratic. Seemingly uncontrollable laughter may develop as well as a voracious appetite that will send the user on an eating binge. Users tend to walk, talk, even sit in peculiar unaccustomed manners. Marijuana reduces motor skills such as those needed for safe driving.

OTHER DANGERS. In the past, marijuana use was termed as a dependence rather than a drug of addiction; however, new research indicates that marijuana is addictive. A great deal of research has also been conducted in relation to the long-term effects of marijuana on the body and mind, and not one study has given marijuana a clean bill of health.

Studies show a person's body tends to develop a tolerance to the drug, so the body still requires larger doses to achieve the same effect. The drug itself seems to lead to the use of harder drugs. Marijuana users lose initiative, ambition, are less productive, and are unable to complete tasks.

HASHISH is a concentrated form of cannabis. Resin from the plant is formed into loaves that are usually dark in color. These loaves (or cakes) are broken up into irregular chunks and sold by the gram. Hashish is five times stronger than marijuana.

COCAINE

COCAINE is derived from the leaves of the coca plant, cultivated in the Andes Mountains in South America. Cocaine enjoyed widespread use in the nineteenth century as a local anesthetic. Cocaine's unique ability to numb as well as inhibit bleeding by constricting blood vessels still makes it an anesthetic popular in nose and throat operations.

Cocaine is processed into a white, crystalline form. In its most popular form, this white flaky powder is bitter, odorless, and numbing to the lips and tongue.

SLANG TERMS. Coke, toot, tootly, blow, snow, candy flake, leaf, C, freeze, happy dust, bernice, bernies, dynamite, flake grin, paradise white, white girl, god dust, speed ball (when mixed with heroin).

METHODS OF ABUSE. Cocaine is sold in powder form. For use it is usually put on a smooth surface, such as a mirror, and cut with a razor blade, fluffing up the powder as well as providing a means of dividing out amounts. "Lines" of cocaine are measured out; each line is then sniffed into a nostril with the aid of a makeshift straw, usually a dollar bill tightly rolled up. This process of "snorting" is the most widespread method of consuming cocaine even though it is sometimes injected directly into the system.

EFFECTS. Cocaine produces a pleasurable body sensation described as an intense adrenaline rush of energy and vigor–may bring feelings of psychic energy, self-confidence, or intense sexuality. It allegedly generates a feeling of renewed strength and endurance. This tends to last about 30 minutes after which the user must again snort to maintain the feelings. Consequently, a great deal of cocaine will be consumed at one sitting, turning a useful and allegedly harmless drug into a dangerous subject.

- Injecting cocaine with unsterile equipment can cause hepatitis or other infections. Furthermore, preparation of free-basing involves the use of volatile solvents, which could cause a fire or explosion, resulting in serious injuries or death. Though few people realize it, overdose deaths can occur when the drug is injected, smoked, or even snorted. Deaths are a result of multiple seizures followed by respiratory and cardiac arrest.

DANGERS. Seemingly pleasant, the stimulating effects of cocaine may escalate into excitability, anxiety, uncontrolled talkativeness, difficulty in focusing the eyes, rapid heartbeat, increased pulse rate, blood pressure elevation, dilated pupils, headaches, nausea, vomiting, increase in body temperature, and hallucinations (particularly that ants or insects are crawling under or on the skin).

Cocaine can also cause lung damage and respiratory problems, distorted thinking, irreversible brain damage, and possible birth defects to the unborn child if used during early pregnancy. Continued use can lead to increased driving accidents, depression, suicide, and death.

COCAINE POISONING. Cold sweats, convulsions, fainting, and a halt in respiration could mean cocaine poisoning has set in which could result in death.

The Multi-Drug Use

A nationwide survey has revealed that those who have or do use cocaine are likely to have used all the other psychoactive drugs, except heroin.

- 100 percent have used alcohol
- 100 percent have used marijuana
- 89 percent psychedelics
- 86 percent stimulants
- 79 percent opiates
- 72 percent sedatives
- 39 percent reported heroin use. The heroin users reported prior use of cocaine.

ALCOHOL

What Is Alcohol?

In medical terms, alcohol is a depressant. It slows the activity of the brain and spinal cord. In chemical terms, alcohol is C_2H_5OH, more commonly known as ethyl alcohol or ethanol. Alcohol is the intoxicating ingredient in alcoholic beverages. Beer and ale contain 4 to 7 percent alcohol; wine contains 9 to 21 percent; and hard liquor contains 40 to 50 percent alcohol.

- The following drinks contain about the same amount of alcohol (1/2 ounce): one 12 oz. can of beer, one 5 oz. glass of wine, one cocktail containing a 1 ½ oz. shot of 86-proof liquor.

Disease

Alcohol, by the effects of its very content, instantly and rapidly affects every organ in the body from the moment the first drink is taken. Alcoholism is a progressive disease. Although patterns and some symptoms can vary, alcoholics progress through basic stages. The disease leads to uncontrollable drinking habits. No single cause has been pin-pointed, although heredity and physiological factors are thought to play a role.

Addiction

Alcoholism is an addiction (dependence), marked by the need to increase doses to produce the desired effect. The body becomes dependent upon the desired effect, and it needs alcohol to function normally. There is also a withdrawal syndrome when alcohol is not taken.

What Does Alcohol Do?

Alcohol enters the bloodstream through the stomach and upper intestine. It circulates rapidly to almost every cell and organ in the body. The central nervous system and the spinal cord are the first parts of the body affected where alcohol acts as a sedative.

Effects of Alcohol on the Brain

Alcohol affects the brain from the outer layers (cortex) to the inner layers (medulla). Once the cortex is affected, the drinker feels the "high" of intoxication. Alcohol can permanently destroy brain cells. Heavy drinking for a long period of time can result in permanent brain damage. Chronic alcoholics can develop a shrinking of the cerebellum, which is a part of the brain that controls equilibrium (balance). This can result in a permanent loss of coordination.

Neuritis

NEURITIS is the inflammation of a nerve. Symptoms of neuritis are tingling, itching, burning, numbness, weakness, and paralysis in the arms and legs.

Delirium Tremens (DTs)

DELIRIUM TREMENS are a violent form of delirium caused by withdrawal from heavy alcohol usage. They are characterized by trembling, sweating, nausea, insomnia, convulsions, delusions, and hallucinations. Ten percent of people who suffer from Delirium Tremens do not survive.

Effect of Alcohol on the Heart

Alcohol weakens the pumping of the heart muscle and decreases the amount of blood to the heart. Alcohol is the most common cause of hypertension (high blood pressure) in the U.S.

WEEK II
DAY 2
ACTIVITY 5:
EXPLORING STIMULANT, DEPRESSANT,
AND NARCOTIC USE

Focus: Physical, psychological effects of stimulants, depressants, and narcotics

Method: Creative drawings/discussion

Time: 1 period

Capsule Description: This exercise is designed to increase the students' awareness of the use of these drugs through creative drawings.

1. Divide the class into three groups: stimulants group, depressants group, narcotics group. Have the students review the substance abuse chart and then brainstorm ways to present information through creative drawings on these types of substances.

2. Provide each group with colored markers and poster paper.

3. At the end of the activity have each group present its information and discuss various ways that the information could be used in a public campaign for substance abuse.

STIMULANTS

STIMULANTS have chemical properties that stimulate (speed up) the actions of the central nervous system. Stimulants are available by prescription for such medical purposes as depression, weight control, narcolepsy (overwhelming attacks of sleep), and hyperactivity in children. According to a national survey, about 20 percent of all medical prescriptions for mood-altering drugs involve stimulants. The drug industry produces enough each year to provide every American citizen with 25 doses. The FDA reports that almost half of this supply enters illegal channels. Many stimulants are also made in makeshift labs.

Amphetamines, commonly called "pep pills," are the most widely known and frequently abused stimulants. They come in various shapes and sizes and their ability to produce increased activity, alertness, and excitation makes them very dangerous to abuse. The drug's effects mask fatigue and abusers exceed their physical endurance without realizing it. Often it is too late. Drivers take them to stay awake on long trips; students use them while cramming for exams; and many criminals use amphetamines to bolster their courage before committing a crime.

Methamphetamine is also a powerful and widely abused stimulant. It has a greater psychological effect than amphetamines and is generally injected.

SLANG TERMS. Pep pills, meth, speed, bennies, uppers, co-pilots, peaches, hearts, wake-ups, sky-rockets, cartwheels, Bomido (injectable form).

METHODS OF ABUSE. Although generally found in pill and capsule form, stimulants are also available in liquid form for injection.

EFFECTS. The consumption of stimulants results in a temporary sense of exhilaration, hyperactivity, loss of appetite, insomnia, extreme amounts of energy, and talkativeness. Stimulant usage produces physical symptoms such as dilated (large) pupils, excessive sweating and body tremors, bad breath, dizziness, dry mouth and lips, and itchy nose. The effects of stimulant abuse can also cause irritability, anxiety, aggressive behavior, panic, and hallucinations. They may cause a sensation known by drug users as a "rush." However when the effects wear off, an unpleasant period of depression called "crashing" follows. All of these effects are greatly intensified when stimulants are taken intravenously. People who take large quantities of stimulants are called "speed freaks."

OTHER DANGERS. Because of the cumulative effects of stimulants, chronic users tend to take "uppers" in the morning to get them going and "downers" in the evening to help them relax and sleep. This can interfere with the normal body processes and can lead to physical and mental illness. Body tolerance develops rapidly and it takes larger doses to achieve the euphoric and appetite suppressant effects, therefore creating DRUG DEPENDENCE. The drug culture has coined a phase: "SPEED KILLS" and eventually it does.

DEPRESSANTS

DEPRESSANTS slow down the body. Their legal use is in the aid of inducing sleep, as sedatives. In low doses, as in tranquilizers, they produce a calming effect on the user. Barbiturates are depressants and when prescribed and monitored by a licensed physician can do much good in relieving sleeplessness and anxiety. However, in excessive amounts depressants produce a state similar to intoxication by alcohol and can lead to addiction, overdosing, and accidents.

Depressants include a wide range of legally prescribable drugs such as Nembutal, Seconal, and Amytal, which are strong barbiturates. Even the so-called "minor tranquilizers," such as Librium, Valium, Equanil, and others used to combat anxiety, can become dangerous, even deadly, when abused. Any depressant in combination with alcohol tends to intensify the likelihood of severe problems. Overdoses result in unconsciousness and death unless there is prompt medical treatment.

SLANG TERMS. Downers, red birds, pines, goofballs, red devils, barbs, candy, peanuts, yellow jackets, yellows.

METHODS OF ABUSE. Depressants come in capsule and tablet form. Some are described as short, intermediate, long-acting and some are time-released. Depressants can be found in liquid form for injection.

EFFECTS. Symptoms of depressant abuse include depression and apathy as well as slurred speech, impaired judgment, and loss of motor coordination. The accompanying disorientation contributes to a high incidence of highway and household accidents among users of depressants. Effects are similar to alcohol intoxication: drowsiness, confusion, tremors, constricted pupils, and depressed blood pressure and respiration. Tolerance to depressants develops rapidly and many abusers will increase the dosage without realizing the dangers.

Depressants are often used by members of the drug culture to reduce the pain from heroin withdrawal, to relieve the anxiety of "flashbacks" resulting from hallucinogenic use, and to soothe the nervous condition brought on by taking stimulants. Combining depressants with alcohol or other drugs greatly increases the danger of abuse.

The main problem with abuse of both depressants and stimulants is their ready availability and the ease of obtaining a prescription for them. Brought on by real ailments, many adults become abusers, by continuing use out of habit, not out of reducing real pain. This type of abuse can cause emotional and physical harm. Depressants are real DOWNERS!

OTHER DANGERS. Depressants, appropriately known as downers, can be addictive. Withdrawal is marked by delirium and convulsions and is especially dangerous. Severe depressant usage can result in cold, clammy skin, weak and rapid pulse, slow and shallow respiration, coma and death.

Symptoms of Abuse

- Drowsiness and lethargy
- Slurred speech and slowed body movements
- "Drifting off" as if in a trance
- Unsteady gait–the appearance of drunkenness without alcohol breath, staggering, and loss of balance
- Quick temper, a quarrelsome disposition
- Faulty judgment
- Depression

NARCOTICS

NARCOTICS in medical terms refer to opium and opium derivatives or synthetic substances. Narcotics are the most effective agents known for the relief of intense pain and are indispensable in medical practice for this purpose. Certain narcotics are used as antidiarrheals; others for respiratory problems. Heroin is the most popular narcotic drug of abuse because of its intense euphoria and long-lasting effects. It has no legitimate use in the United States. Heroin is synthesized from morphine and is ten times as potent. It is a bitter-tasting powder which varies in color from white to dark brown. Pure heroin is rarely sold on the street since traffickers "cut" or dilute heroin so that the substance sold contains less than five percent heroin. The use of narcotics generates physical dependence, addiction, and an increased tolerance to the drug.

NARCOTIC NAMES. Opium, Morphine, Codeine, Heroin, Hydromorphone, Diluadid, Methadone, Lomotil, and Percodan. Cocaine also is classified as a narcotic.

SLANG TERMS. Horse, H, Smack, Boy, White Stuff, Harry, Junk, Hard Stuff, Miss Emma, Morpho, M, Unkie, Dollies, Cotics, Dope.

METHODS OF ABUSE. Heroin is usually injected directly into the bloodstream by the abuser (mainlining). It also can be administered under the skin (skin-popping), or snorted like cocaine. Some narcotics are available in tablet and capsule form.

EFFECTS. The euphoric effects of narcotics are short-lived. The subsequent effects are pinpoint pupils, reduced vision, drowsiness, apathy, decreased physical activity, constipation, sleep, nausea, vomiting, and respiratory depression.

BLACK TAR HEROIN

Sometimes known as "Tootsie Roll," "Goma," and a variety of other street names, including just plain "junk," Black Tar is smuggled into the States primarily by illegal aliens and migrant workers.

APPEARANCE. May appear dark brown to black in color. It may be sticky like roofing tar or hard like coal. It is readily moisture-absorbent and will appear to melt in the presence of heat or humidity. It is generally water-soluble except for its contaminants, opium by-products which are not removed during initial processing. Black Tar has a repulsive vinegar-like odor which becomes noticeable two to five hours after processing or when exposed to the air for a length of time.

METHODS OF ABUSE. Most commonly injected; however, users have snorted and smoked Black Tar with varied results.

Symptoms of Abuse

- Long scars, like tattoos, along veins. These are caused by veins collapsing from the continual injection of narcotics
- Equipment–spoon bent for the purpose of cooking substance to injection consistency; syringe and needle, can be store-bought, but most often homemade; strap or belt for raising the vein
- Marks on body–punctures (tracks) from injecting, black and blue marks from skin-popping
- Lethargic and indifferent to surroundings

WITHDRAWAL SYMPTOMS. Withdrawing from narcotics begins shortly before the time of the next scheduled dose. The intensity of physical symptoms is directly related to the amount of the drug used each day.

Total physical withdrawal for an addict lasts seven to ten days and the symptoms are: runny nose, watery eyes, perspiration, yawning, restlessness, irritability, loss of appetite, insomnia, body tremors, nausea, vomiting, stomach cramps, diarrhea, panic, chills, pain, and muscle spasms.

OTHER DANGERS. Addicts risk hepatitis, AIDS, and infection from using contaminated needles. Since purity is difficult to determine, potency is unpredictable. For this reason overdoses resulting in death are common. Physical dependence on narcotics necessitates the need to have a continuous presence of the drug in the body to prevent the withdrawal symptoms.

Repeated use of narcotics results in increased tolerance, therefore requiring larger amounts to achieve the desired effect. DRUG DEPENDENCE most likely will occur.

WEEK II
DAY 3
ACTIVITY 6:
EXPLORING HALLUCINOGEN AND INHALANT USE

Focus: Physical and psychological effects of hallucinogens and inhalants

Method: Worksheet/discussion

Time: 1 period

Capsule Description: This exercise is designed to increase the students' awareness of hallucinogen and inhalant use.

1. Using the substance abuse chart, review with the class information related to hallucinogens and inhalants.

2. Divide the class into pairs. Give each pair a photocopied list of statements with multiple choice answers. Have each pair read the statements and select the best possible answer.

3. Reconvene the class, present the statements, and solicit the responses from all pairs. Compare the responses given to the list of correct responses.

4. Have the students discuss their reactions to the exercise.

LIST OF STATEMENTS
FOR HALLUCINOGENS/INHALANT ACTIVITY

Directions: Read the following statements and circle the correct answer(s).

1. Certain common name(s) for hallucinogens are:
   A. PCP   B. Snow   C. Ecstasy   D. LSD   E. Uppers

2. A possible effect(s) of hallucinogens are:
   A. Dilated pupils   C. Slurred or blocked speech
   B. Death   D. Hallucinations   E. Psychosis

3. During the 1970s, _____ deaths occurred as a result of sniffing Freon aerosol in vegetable spray.
   A. 24   B. 1500   C. 67   D. 700   E. 219

4. LSD has been found in/on:
   A. Sugar cubes   B. Candy   C. Liquor
   D. Aspirin   E. Back of postage stamps

5. Symptoms of inhalant abuse include:
   A. Nosebleeds   D. Nausea
   B. Slow heartbeat   E. Increased hand/eye coordination
   C. Feeling and looking tired

6. Overdoses of inhalants produce:
   A. Damage to lungs, kidneys, liver, and bone marrow
   B. Suffocation   D. Brain damage
   C. Sudden death   E. Stroke

7. PCP is used medically for:
   A. Adults   D. Monkeys
   B. Children   E. Horses
   C. Cancer patients

8. After taking LSD, hallucinations may recur:
   A. Only if it is used again   D. Months later
   B. Within 24 hours   E. For an unknown amount of time
   C. Days later

9. People who start with inhalants and go on to other drugs usually:
   A. Stop using inhalants   B. Cut down on inhalants

10. If inhalant usage is mixed with other drugs:
    A. Loss of consciousness may occur   C. Coma may occur
    B. Nothing happens   D. Death is possible

Answers for Hallucinogens/Inhalant Activity

1. A,C,D   6. A,B,C,D,E
2. A,B,C,D,E   7. D,E
3. D   8. A,B,C,D,E
4. A,B,C,D,E   9. B
5. A,C,D   10. A,C,D

WEEK II
DAY 4
TEAM PRACTICE SESSION

Focus: Preparation for TGT tournament
Method: Worksheets
Time: 1 period
Capsule Description: The students work in their TGT teams on specially prepared worksheets in preparation for the TGT tournament.

Divide the class members into their TGT teams and let them work the worksheets in their small groups. Instruct the groups to discuss each question, coming to a consensus answer for each question. Circulate through the class to check the groups' progress and answer any questions. When all groups are finished with the worksheets, go over them as a class and provide them with correct answers so that they may study for the tournament tomorrow.

TEAM WORKSHEET II

1. True or False: Cellular damage from marijuana is a proven fact.

2. A form of amnesia, lasting from seconds to days, resulting from alcohol use is a _____ .

3. The effects of stimulant abuse can cause:
   A. aggressive behavior   B. panic   C. hallucination

4. True or False: Depressants used in combination with alcohol can cause death.

5. _____ is the most widespread method of using cocaine.

6. True or False: The repeated use of narcotics results in decreased tolerance.

7. True or False: Moderate to heavy marijuana use by males results in a decreased sperm count and an abundance of abnormally formed sperm.

8. Name three types of inhalants.

9. True or False: Withdrawal from depressants, although physically uncomfortable, is not dangerous.

10. The effects of cocaine last about _____ minutes. Therefore, a great deal of cocaine will be consumed at one sitting, leading to dangers that can result in cold sweats, convulsions, fainting, a halt in respiration, and possible death.

11. True or False: Alcohol instantly and rapidly affects every organ in the body from the moment the first drink is taken.

12. _____, commonly called "pep pills," are the most widely known and frequently abused stimulants.

13. True or False: The unseen danger of marijuana is the possibility of substances, such as PCP or cocaine, being sprayed on the leaves to enhance the marijuana or obtain another type of high.

14. _____ is synthesized from morphine and is ten times as potent.

15. Anxiety, an incapacitating tenseness, and suicidal tendencies may persist for weeks or months following withdrawal from _____ .

16. Crack is a _____ and users often become intensely active, frequently exhibiting signs of paranoia. Dependency can occur in as little as two weeks.

17. True or False: The intravenous injection of narcotics or other substances can result in hepatitis, AIDS, or infection from contaminated needles.

18. True or False: The effects of marijuana on female reproduction are of short duration.

19. Heavy drinking for a long period of time can result in (permanent/temporary) brain damage.

20. True or False: Studies have shown that chronic exposure to some solvents and gasoline causes leukemia and severe anemia.

21. _____ is the most common contaminant found in a number of street drugs.
    A. PCP   B. codeine   C. heroin   D. crack

ANSWERS TO TEAM WORKSHEET II

1. True
2. Blackout
3. A,B,C
4. True
5. Snorting
6. False
7. True
8. Possible answers: gasoline, deodorant, airplane glue, vegetable spray, hair spray, spray paint, liquid paper, paint thinner, rubber cement
9. False
10. 30 to 120
11. True
12. Amphetamines
13. True
14. Heroin
15. Stimulants
16. Stimulant
17. True
18. False
19. Permanent
20. True
21. A

WEEK II
DAY 5
TOURNAMENT

Focus: Summarizing, integrating week's activities
Method: Game
Time: 1 period
Capsule Description: Students in their TGT teams compete for points by correctly answering questions based on the week's activities.

Divide the class into the tournament tables. Go over the rules of play again and the "GIGS" if students need reminding. Pass out Game B, Game B Answer sheet, and Game Score Sheet to each team. Answer any questions. At the end of the tournament, fill out the Team Summary Sheet, Tournament Score Sheet, and publicize the results. Then devise new tournament tables according to the "bumping" procedure.

GAME B
EXPLORING PSYCHOACTIVE SUBSTANCE USE

B-1   The effects of cocaine last about how many minutes?

B-2   True or False: The repeated use of narcotics results in increased tolerance.

B-3   What is the danger for males using marijuana in moderate to heavy levels?

B-4   What are two disorders that result from chronic exposures to solvents and gasoline?

B-5   Intravenous injections with contaminated needles can result in what type of infections?

B-6   True or False: PCP is the most common contaminant found in a number of street drugs.

B-7   What is a form of amnesia, lasting from seconds to days, resulting from alcohol use?

B-8   Name one effect of stimulant abuse.

B-9   What classification of drugs used in combination with alcohol can cause death?

B-10   True or False: Withdrawal from depressants, although physically uncomfortable, is not dangerous.

B-11   Deodorant, vegetable sprays, and gasoline belong to which drug classification?

B-12   True or False: Snorting is the most widespread method of using cocaine.

B-13   Anxiety, an incapacitating tenseness, and suicidal tendencies may persist for weeks or months following withdrawal from what classification of drugs?

B-14   What drug has been proven to cause cellular damage?

B-15   True or False: Persons cannot become dependent on crack.

B-16   True or False: Heavy drinking for a long period of time can result in permanent brain damage.

B-17   What are the most widely abused stimulants?

B-18   What is synthesized from morphine and is ten times as potent?

B-19   True or False: Marijuana has long-term effects on female reproduction.

B-20   Crack users frequently exhibit what type of psychological disturbance?

B-21   True or False: The unseen danger of marijuana is the possibility of substances such as PCP, heroin, or cocaine being sprayed on the leaves.

B-22 After taking LSD, hallucinations may recur for how long?

B-23 True or False: If inhalant usage occurs with other drug use, death may occur.

GAME B ANSWER SHEET
EXPLORING PSYCHOACTIVE SUBSTANCE USE

B-1 30 to 120
B-2 True
B-3 Decreased sperm count and an abundance of abnormally formed sperm
B-4 Anemia and leukemia
B-5 Hepatitis, AIDS
B-6 True
B-7 Blackouts
B-8 Aggressive behavior or panic or hallucinations
B-9 Depressants
B-10 False
B-11 Organic solvents
B-12 True
B-13 Stimulants
B-14 Marijuana
B-15 False
B-16 True
B-17 Amphetamines or pep pills
B-18 Heroin
B-19 True
B-20 Paranoia
B-21 True
B-22 Months later or even longer
B-23 True

WEEK III
DAY 1
ACTIVITY 7:
THE PHYSICAL EFFECTS OF PSYCHOACTIVE
SUBSTANCE USE AND ATTITUDES TOWARD USE

Focus: Prevalence of substance abuse
Method: Poll/discussion
Time: 1-2 periods
Capsule Description: This exercise is designed to introduce students to others' substance use practices and to serve as a springboard for students learning of the relationship between attitudes toward substance use. Students design and administer to others a poll to measure their attitudes and reasons for using or not using psychoactive substances.

1. Have your students divide up into small groups and brainstorm their own questions to gauge how much and how often people use substances and in what situations they use, why people use or abstain, and their attitudes toward using and not using. Sample questions are provided at the end of this activity which may be used as examples or comparisons. Following the small group brainstorming, the class as a whole can then develop a single master questionnaire incorporating the best questions from each group's poll.

2. In small groups or as a class, have students administer the poll anonymously to other people, such as students, school faculty, parents, or others. One group of students can be responsible for polling students, one group for polling faculty, etc.

3. Have each group of students tabulate the results and present them to the class. Discuss what was learned, and compare the actual results with what students thought the poll would reveal.

4. Sample poll questions:

   a. Have you ever used any psychoactive substances for non-medicinal purposes? (circle one)
       Yes   No

   b. When you drink or use drugs for nonmedicinal purposes it is usually:
      alone   with others   never used

c. How old were you when you had your first drink (that is, one full glass of wine, one can or bottle of beer, one mixed drink or shot of liquor)?
under 8 9 10 11 12 13 14 15 16 17 18 19 20
over 20   do not remember   never used

d. How old were you when you used a psychoactive substance nonmedicinally?
under 8 9 10 11 12 13 14 15 16 17 18 19 20
over 20   do not remember   never used

e. Where and with whom did you have your first drink or nonmedicinal psychoactive substance? (circle one)

with parents	with relatives	with friends
at home	at a friend's home	at a relative's
in a car	in a restaurant	in school
alone	other	never used

f. Have you ever felt others put pressure on you to drink or use non-medicinal drugs?
                    Yes   No

g. If you drink or use drugs for nonmedicinal purposes, for which of the following purposes?

to relax	to be sociable	to get drunk	to do what
to forget	to get high	for religious	my friends
worries	to be different	reasons	are doing
to act grown	to enjoy the	to quench my	for kicks
up	taste	thirst	other
to celebrate			

h. If you do not drink or use drugs for nonmedicinal purposes, for which of the following reasons do you not?

do not like the taste	my friends do not drink/use
like to be different	just am not interested
alcohol/drugs make me sick	believe it is wrong
against my religion	drinking/drugs look bad
too expensive	other

i. Which, if any, are good reasons to drink or use drugs in moderation?

escape problems	taste	kicks
relieve nervousness	pressure from	to relax
tradition	friend	to feel mature
be sociable	religious	to get high
celebration	ceremonies	other

j. What do you think about drinking/psychoactive drugs and driving?

would never do it

would do it to get home on time

would do it in an emergency

would do it if I knew I would not get caught

would not ride with anyone who had been drinking/using drugs

would try to arrange another ride home

5. Sample follow-up questions you can ask the students after they have administered the questionnaires:

a. What types of influence might affect people's substance use behavior?

b. Does the poll show any difference between the way men and women use these substances differently? How? Why?

c. What are the most common reasons people give for using or abstaining from psychoactive substances? Do different groups give different reasons (for example, teachers compared to students)?

d. Do you think your questions were answered honestly? If not, why do you think some people were reluctant? What does this say about the role of psychoactive substances in our society?

e. What seems to be the most common attitude toward using psychoactive substances? Did different groups express different attitudes? If so, what might explain the difference?

f. Do students feel that any of the attitudes expressed in the poll were inappropriate? Why?

g. How does the class think people develop attitudes toward psychoactive substances? Can attitudes toward using or abstaining change? What influences does the class think could change attitudes toward using or not using?

h. What was the most common attitude expressed about using psychoactive substances and driving? What reasons did people give for their decisions?

WEEK III
DAY 2
ACTIVITY 8:
SURFACING AND EXPLORING ATTITUDES ABOUT PSYCHOACTIVE SUBSTANCES

Focus: Attitudes
Method: Discussion
Time: 1 period
Capsule Description: Students engage in activities designed to surface, explore, and increase their awareness as to their own feelings about using psychoactive substances or not using them. Five brief mini-activities follow that can be used singularly or in combination to help your students identify their attitudes toward psychoactive substances so that they can compare and discuss their feelings toward using and not using.

1. Interpreting Pictures of Psychoactive Substance Use

Supply your students with photographs or drawings from magazines which depict some type of substance-using behavior. Cut off any captions or explanations of the materials but number the captions and the pictures so that they may be reunited later.

Give each student a picture and have them write what they think is occurring in the picture and why substance use is taking place.

After each picture is discussed, read the corresponding caption and discuss how the picture was accurately assessed or why they may have misinterpreted the picture.

Finally, make a list on the blackboard of the reasons the students gave why people use substances.

2. Analyzing Humor About Psychoactive Substance Use

This exercise is similar to interpreting pictures. Supply the students with cartoons, jokes, comic strips or greeting cards that involve psychoactive substance usage in some manner. Break the class into small groups and give them written instructions to:

a. examine the materials
b. list the reasons stated or implied why the individuals in the cartoons, etc., are using substances
c. decide and record your attitudes about the using behavior

Have the group report their findings to the class and compare and discuss the results.

3. Examining Songs About Psychoactive Substance Use

Break your class into groups and have them collect records, lyrics, or tape recordings of songs that describe substance usage. Have each group select one song to present to the class. Have the class identify what attitudes toward using are expressed in each song and whether these attitudes are "healthy" ones or not and why. Have the group members identify why they chose to present that particular song.

4. Psychoactive Substance Use on Special Occasions

Ask your students to brainstorm the "special occasions" when alcohol or other psychoactive substances are provided. Ask the students to offer their suggestions and write them on the board. When major occasions have been identified, discuss the categories of occasions represented–celebrations, religious ceremonies, parties, etc. Note the different types of events where alcohol/drugs would be present for some groups and not for others (example: most Jewish families serve alcohol at weddings; many Christian families do not; certain Indian tribes use hallucinogens during rituals, etc.).

Select one event where alcohol is usually served and ask the class if everyone who attends such an event would drink and why. Then select an event at which drinking would probably not occur and discuss why.

Tell the class to look for occasions in the next week–special and ordinary events–at which drinking/drug use takes place and to think about why psychoactive substances are served at them. The occasions can take place in their homes, on television, or among their friends or parents' friends.

5. Pluses and Minuses of Psychoactive Substance Use

Have the students brainstorm on the blackboard all the benefits of substance use on one side and all the negative aspects of substance use on the other. Have students cite observations they have noted which lead them to their ideas–from observing friends, relatives, TV shows, etc.

WEEK III
DAY 3
ACTIVITY 9
PHYSICAL AND BEHAVIORAL EFFECTS
OF PSYCHOACTIVE SUBSTANCES

Focus: Physical effects of psychoactive substance
Method: Diagram
Time: 1/2 period
Capsule Description: Students trace the passage of psychoactive substances through the body on a specially prepared body diagram. Pass out copies of the blank body chart provided on the following page (they may be mimeographed or photocopied) and have your students try to identify what the body organs are that are displayed. Review the organs and their major functions. Then ask your students to draw, to the best of their knowledge, the paths that psychoactive substances follow as they pass through the body. It may be helpful to break the class into groups of three or four, have them do the diagram as a group and compare results between groups.

After the class has had a chance to indicate how it thinks psychoactive substances pass through the body, pass out copies of the filled-in body diagram. Review with the class the correct steps in the passage of psychoactive substances through the body.

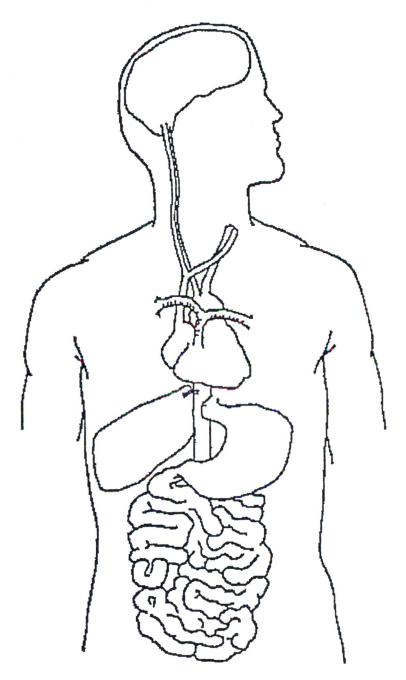

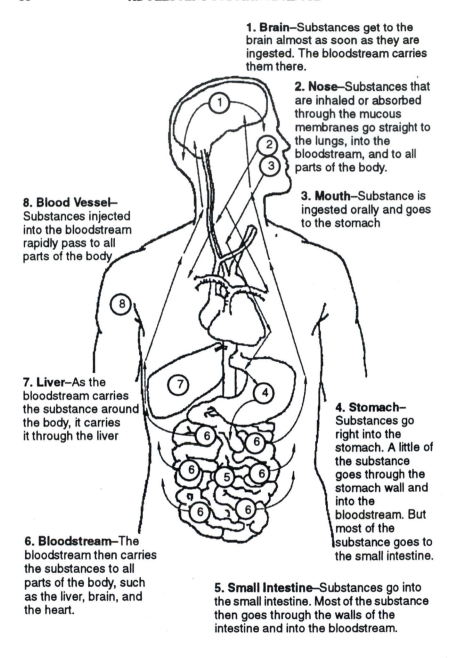

1. Brain–Substances get to the brain almost as soon as they are ingested. The bloodstream carries them there.

2. Nose–Substances that are inhaled or absorbed through the mucous membranes go straight to the lungs, into the bloodstream, and to all parts of the body.

3. Mouth–Substance is ingested orally and goes to the stomach

8. Blood Vessel–Substances injected into the bloodstream rapidly pass to all parts of the body

7. Liver–As the bloodstream carries the substance around the body, it carries it through the liver

4. Stomach–Substances go right into the stomach. A little of the substance goes through the stomach wall and into the bloodstream. But most of the substance goes to the small intestine.

6. Bloodstream–The bloodstream then carries the substances to all parts of the body, such as the liver, brain, and the heart.

5. Small Intestine–Substances go into the small intestine. Most of the substance then goes through the walls of the intestine and into the bloodstream.

WEEK III
DAY 3
ACTIVITY 10:
ALCOHOL'S PHYSICAL AND BEHAVIORAL EFFECTS

Focus: Effects of alcohol on the body
Method: Discussion/Mini-lecture
Time: 1/4 - 1/2 period
Capsule Description: Following a mini-lecture, students discuss alcohol's effects on the mind and body. Although we feel students will learn and retain more information about alcohol through role play, small group discussion, and independent study, a mini-lecture about some physical effects of alcohol is used here as a reinforce-able introduction to the subject area. Categorized below are the major topics you might want to cover in a mini-lecture on alcohol.

Even though alcohol passes through everyone's body the same way, there are several factors which determine what effects the alcohol will have. These are:

1. how much the person drinks
2. how fast the person drinks
3. what kind of alcoholic beverage is drunk
4. how much the person weighs
5. how much the person has eaten
6. the state or condition of the body
7. how the person thinks and feels about drinking
8. where a person drinks–the setting

1. Amount of Alcohol

The most important influence on how alcohol affects a person is how much alcohol is drunk. The more alcohol, the greater the effects.

Contrary to popular opinions, whiskey is not "stronger" than beer or wine. 5 oz. wine = 12 oz. can of beer = 1½ shot of whiskey

2. Speed of Drinking

The liver metabolizes alcohol (converts it to carbon dioxide and water) at the steady rate of 3/4 ounce in an hour; it circulates in the bloodstream until the liver can metabolize it. During this process of circulation, the alcohol keeps passing through the brain. Consequently, the faster alcohol is drunk, the more alcohol reaches the brain (and other body organs), producing faster, more potent effects on the drinker.

3. Type of Beverage Consumed

Liquor is absorbed more readily than either beer or wine, and combining liquor with carbonated drinks will increase the rate even more. Water, on the other hand, dilutes alcohol and slows down the rate.

4. Body Weight

People who weigh more are affected less by alcohol than lighter people. Heavier people have more blood and water in their bodies to diffuse the alcohol.

5. Food

Food slows down the passage of alcohol through the stomach. Consequently, alcohol will "go to your head" if you have not eaten before drinking or eat while you drink.

6. Body Condition

A drinker who is tired may be more influenced by the alcohol drunk than a person who is alert. An ill person may be more affected than a healthy person. Especially worthwhile to note is that alcohol plus other drugs are not simply addictive–they are multiplicative. Alcohol can have double or triple its normal sedative effects when mixed with other drugs.

7. Thoughts and Feelings About Drinking

Experienced drinkers often develop a psychological tolerance for alcohol. On the basis of many drinking experiences, they have learned what effects alcohol has on them and can compensate for them. Along this same line, alcohol often affects a person the way he or she expects it to. When drinkers expect to get high, they are likely to do so. Also, a person's mood affects what alcohol does to them. Alcohol may make someone who is feeling unhappy more depressed, or someone cheerful even happier. Finally, where someone drinks–the setting–may affect how much they drink and how alcohol affects them. A person might drink moderately away from friends and feel the effects whereas at a tense gathering may not feel the effects as readily.

WEEK III
DAY 4
TEAM PRACTICE SESSION

Focus: Preparation for TGT tournament
Method: Worksheets
Time: 1 period
Capsule Description: The students work in their TGT teams on specially prepared worksheets in preparation for the TGT tournament.

Divide the class members into their TGT teams and let them complete the worksheets in their small groups. Instruct the groups to discuss each question, coming to a consensus answer for each question. Circulate through the class to check the groups' progress and answer any questions. When all groups are finished with worksheets, go over them as a class and provide them with correct answers so that they may study for the tournament tomorrow.

TEAM WORKSHEET III

1. Name three common reasons people give for using psychoactive substances.

2. Name three common reasons people give for not using psychoactive substances.

3. Name one way a person develops his/her attitude toward using psychoactive substances.

4. True or False: Many people use psychoactive substances as a way to be with friends socially.

5. True or False: Psychoactive substances are only used in the U.S. and parts of Europe–they have not been used much by other cultures.

6. True or False: Alcohol is the most commonly used psychoactive substance consumed by Americans.

7. True or False: The media has a big impact on how people view using psychoactive substances.

8. When a psychoactive substances is ingested, the first organ it goes to is the _____ .

9. When psychoactive substances are snorted or inhaled, they go directly to the _____ .

10. The liver metabolizes alcohol at what rate?

11. How much wine equals one 12 oz. glass of beer?

12. Psychoactive substances get to the _____ almost as soon as they are ingested.

13. List three settings where psychoactive substance use may occur.

14. Why is it good to serve food when serving alcohol at a party?

15. Give three reasons for not using psychoactive substances and driving.

16. Once psychoactive substances enter the brain, do they stay there or circulate back through the body again?

17. True or False: Drinking liquor with soda pop will increase the rate at which it is absorbed into the bloodstream.

18. The _____ metabolizes psychoactive substances.

19. True or False: According to the National Academy of Sciences, the National Institute on Alcohol Abuse and Alcoholism, and the National Institute on Drug Abuse, 100,000 to 120,000 deaths annually are directly attributable to substance abuse.

20. True or False: More teenagers die in drug and alcohol-related motor vehicle accidents than from any disease.

ANSWERS TO TEAM WORKSHEET III

1. Examples of answers: to relax, be social, it tastes good, my friends do, to celebrate special occasions, to get high, to be different, to have a good time.

2. Examples of answers: do not believe in it, religion is against it, just not interested, do not like the taste, to be different, it is wrong.

3. Watching parents, the community in which he/she lives, being around friends, deciding for him/herself.

4. True

5. False

6. True

7. True

8. Stomach

9. Lungs

10. 3/4 oz. per hour

11. 5 oz. wine = 12 oz. beer

12. Bloodstream

13. Parties, out with friends, while alone, at school, recreational parks.

14. Because it slows down the absorption rate of alcohol into the bloodstream and keeps a person from getting light-headed.

15. Might injure self, might injure others, might damage property, might damage car.

16. Circulate back through the body.

17. True

18. Liver

19. True

20. True

WEEK III
DAY 5
TOURNAMENT

Focus: Summarizing, integrating week's activities
Method: Game
Time: 1 period
Capsule Description: Students in their TGT teams compete for points by correctly answering questions based on the week's activities.

Divide the class into the tournament tables. Go over the rules of play again and the "GIGS" if students need reminding. Pass out Game C, Game C Answer Sheet, and Game Score Sheet to each team. Answer any questions. At the end of the tournament, fill out the Team Summary Sheet, Tournament Score Sheet, and publicize the results. Then devise new tournament tables according to the "bumping" procedure.

GAME C
THE PHYSICAL EFFECTS OF PSYCHOACTIVE
SUBSTANCE USE AND ATTITUDES TOWARD USE

C-1   What organs do psychoactive substances go to when snorted or inhaled?

C-2   What are some reasons people give for not using psychoactive substances?

C-3   True or False: Eating while drinking alcohol slows down the absorption rate of alcohol in the bloodstream.

C-4   Do only a few select cultures use psychoactive substances?

C-5   True or False: People use psychoactive substances to relax or to be social.

C-6   What is the most common psychoactive substance used by Americans?

C-7   How many deaths each year are directly attributable to substance abuse?

C-8   True or False: The kidneys metabolize psychoactive substances.

C-9   Could a person's attitude toward using psychoactive substances be influenced by his/her community's attitudes?

C-10   True or False: For teenagers, the number of substance abuse deaths are greater than motor vehicle deaths.

C-11   A 12 oz. beer equals how much wine?

C-12   The liver metabolizes alcohol at what rate?

C-13   What is a possible consequence of using psychoactive substances and driving?

C-14   True or False: Drinking liquor with soda pop will decrease the rate alcohol is absorbed into the bloodstream.

C-15   What is the first organ that a psychoactive substance goes to once it is ingested?

C-16   True or False: Many people use psychoactive substances as a way to interact with friends socially.

C-17   After entering the brain, do psychoactive substances circulate through the body again?

C-18   How quickly do psychoactive substances enter the bloodstream?

C-19   Can the media influence drug-using behavior?

C-20   What are two settings where psychoactive substance use typically occurs?

C-21   True or False: A person's body condition can influence the effect that psychoactive substance use may have on him/her.

C-22   Can a person's expectations about the effects of alcohol make a difference in how alcohol will affect him/her?

GAME C ANSWER SHEET
THE PHYSICAL EFFECTS OF PSYCHOACTIVE
SUBSTANCE USE AND ATTITUDES TOWARD USE

C-1   Lungs
C-2   Do not believe in it, religion is against it, just not interested, do not like the taste, to be different, it is wrong
C-3   True
C-4   No
C-5   True
C-6   Alcohol
C-7   100,000 to 120,000
C-8   False
C-9   Yes
C-10   True
C-11   5 oz. wine
C-12   3/4 oz. per hour

C-13   Injury to self or to others, damage to car or property, legal charges
C-14   False
C-15   Stomach
C-16   True
C-17   Yes
C-18   Almost as soon as they are ingested
C-19   Yes
C-20   At parties, with friends
C-21   True
C-22   Yes

WEEK IV
DAY 1
ACTIVITY 11:
PSYCHOACTIVE SUBSTANCE USE DECISIONS
AND PEER PRESSURE

Focus: Substance abuse
Method: Group discussion
Time: 1/2 period
Capsule Description: Students discuss and decide what they think constitutes substance abuse.

Break your class into small groups and have them brainstorm the characteristics and behavior of someone who uses mood-altering substances. Have the students construct a list of the behaviors they have identified in their small groups. When the small groups have finished, try to see if the class can reach a consensus on substance abuse behaviors. Each group can present its decisions and following discussion, these behaviors can be listed on the blackboard. A point to review with students: our society has been one that has sanctioned the use of psychoactive substances to alleviate psychological as well as physical discomfort. Have the students discuss when use becomes abuse. For example, taking more than the prescribed dosage–"if one makes you feel good, two will make you feel great"; taking drugs prescribed for a peer, parent, or other; drinking to escape from problems or to build confidence.

WEEK IV
DAY 1
ACTIVITY 12:
SUBSTANCE ABUSE WORD GAMES

Focus: Effects of substance abuse
Method: Games
Time: 1/2 period
Capsule Description: Students develop and play word games in which psychoactive substance terms are used and defined. Several word games are presented on the following pages which students may play individually or in small groups.
1. Unscrambling Words
   One student thinks of a substance abuse term and writes on the board with the letters scrambled. The other students unscramble the term but must define it when they have figured it out.
   Examples:

       ecoinca–cocaine   aculhailinont-hallucination
       rzieuse–seizure   ocalhlo–alcohol
       iarmjaanu–marijuana

2. Substance Abuse Word Link
   Fill in the missing letters in the substance abuse related words listed below.

____R____ CK   ____S____
____ L____ OHL   ____OX____ ____
____A___G___R   ____N___ALE
              DEL____RIU____

Now rearrange the letters you filled in to spell the name of the condition that can result from the repeated use of psychoactive substances.

__ __ __ __ __ __ __ __ __ __ __ __ __ __ __ __ __

Answers : Crack, LSD, Alcohol, Toxic, Danger, Inhale, Delirium.
Condition: Chemical Addiction.

WEEK IV
DAY 2
ACTIVITY 13:
IS SUBSTANCE ABUSE OK?

Focus: Reasons for using psychoactive substances
Method: Discussion
Time: 1 period
Capsule Description: Students discuss whether and when it might be appropriate to use psychoactive substances.

Have your students break into small groups. Provide each group with a different scenario and instruct them to discuss whether using psychoactive substances in that particular situation is all right, and why or why not. Have the groups come to a consensus on their decision. When all groups have completed the exercise, have each group report to the class its decision and why. Encourage close discussion of the decision. Here are some considerations that students may want to explore:

- Is it effective in the long run not to face and solve problems?
- Is it all right not to face problems that are temporary or cannot be solved? In deciding whether using is all right or not, the students may want to discuss within their groups:
    a. How many times is the person going to use the substance as an escape?
    b. How much is he or she suffering?
    c. How much will his or her use hurt him/herself or others?
    d. Is the problem soluble if confronted, or insoluble?
    e. Is the person using with full awareness of possible consequences?

Sample Scenarios

- A person's steady date insists that the person snort cocaine with him/her. Is it OK to use once? Whenever the steady insists? Why or why not?
- A mother feels depressed following her divorce. Is it OK for her to take prescribed antidepressants? Should she take more than recommended? Should she give one to a friend who is depressed? Why or why not?

• A woman drives to a party and drinks a great deal of alcohol while smoking marijuana. Is it OK for her to drive home after drinking a strong cup of coffee? Why or why not?

WEEK IV
DAY 3
ACTIVITY 13:
PEER PRESSURE TO USE PSYCHOACTIVE SUBSTANCES

Focus: Peer Pressure
Method: Letter Writing/Role Play
Time: 1 period
Capsule Description: Students engage in an activity revolving around peer pressure to abstain, use, or use abusively.

This activity has two options: you might want to use them separately or in conjunction with one another. Have the class break into small groups.

Option 1

Have your students explore ways to cope with peer pressure to use or abstain by responding to hypothetical letters (in "Dear Abby" fashion) from various age students in situations of conflict about substance use. Sample letters are provided below. Students can write or present verbally the answers to the letters. If the students in the groups disagree with each other about what the "advice" should be, they may draft more than one letter. Follow-up discussion with the entire class could center around how different approaches may be most useful for different people on different occasions.

Option 2

Your students can also role play scenes in which someone is being pressured to use, use excessively, or abstain. Sample role profiles are provided at the end of the activity. Follow-up discussion can center on what techniques seemed to be effective in resisting pressure, how people feel about using drugs or alcohol, and why people try to exert pressure on others to use, use excessively, or abstain.

Option 1: Sample "Dear Abby" Letters

Dear Abby,

I'm 13 years old and sometimes when I go out with my three best friends they get an older brother to buy us some marijuana. Usually someone's parents are out and we go over to their house and smoke. My friends get pretty high sometimes. I try to inhale as little as possible without their noticing, but they do, and pressure me to inhale as deeply as they inhale. I am afraid of getting high and losing control and my parents finding out. I'm not interested in smoking marijuana, but these are my three closest friends. What do I do?

Unsure

* * *

Dear Abby,

Last week I went to the movies with three friends. On the way home we ran into some older kids; one of them was a guy I would like to date. They gave us some kind of white pill saying, "This will give you a great high. If you're really grown up, you will try it." I didn't want any because I didn't know what it was and what it might do. Now the kids at school call me chicken and say that I'm a baby. I don't like being picked on by my friends and now I feel that I've blown it with that guy. What can I do?

Bothered

* * *

Dear Abby,

A couple of weeks ago a guy I know from school came by my house and asked if I wanted to go and play some video games. He had his dad's car for a couple of hours. As soon as we drove off, my friend pulled a beer out from under the seat and offered me some. I took a sip and he drank the rest of it. He also snorted some cocaine. By the time we got to the game center he was acting kind of crazy and while we played games he kept going back out to the car. I was kind of afraid to ride home with him, but I was afraid to call my parents and ask them to come and get me because they are always acting suspicious of my friends anyway. What should I have done?

Afraid

Option 2: Sample Role Profiles

User: You are at a friend's house but nobody is home. Your friend's parents are out for the evening. You obtained some marijuana from an older cousin and neither you nor your friend have ever used it. You want to try some–you do not think anyone will ever find out. How will you be able to persuade your friend to try some?

Friend: You have invited a friend over because your parents are out for the night. Your friend has brought some marijuana–neither one of you have ever tried it. Your parents have trusted you and you know they would be angry and disappointed if you used pot. Your friend wants to smoke the marijuana, but you are afraid. What do you say to let your friend know you do not want to?

Friend #2: You have been out with a gang of your friends playing video games and eating pizza. Some older kids ride by and ask if you and your friends would like to go "party" with them. You are supposed to be home in half an hour and are not sure about going off with the other kids–you have heard they are pretty wild and experiment with drugs. You refuse but most of your friends go. The next day when you see them, they give you a hard time about not going. What do you do?

WEEK IV
DAY 4
TEAM PRACTICE SESSION

Focus: Preparation for TGT tournament
Method: Worksheets
Time: 1 period
Capsule Description: The students work in their TGT teams on specially prepared worksheets in preparation for the TGT tournament.

Divide the class into their TGT teams and let them work the worksheets in these small groups. Instruct the class to discuss each question as a group, coming to a consensus answer for each question. Circulate through the class to check the group's progress and answer any questions. When all groups are finished with the worksheets, go over them as a class and provide them with correct answers so if they like that they may study for the tournament tomorrow.

TEAM WORKSHEET IV

1. True or False: American society has sanctioned the use of psychoactive substances prescribed by physicians to alleviate emotional discomfort.

2. Name three negative consequences of abusing psychoactive substances.

3. True or False: It is okay to take medication prescribed for someone else if you have similar symptoms.

4. Unscramble this word: ECOINCA

5. True or False: Everyone has to decide for him or herself if and how much he/she will use psychoactive substances.

6. Unscramble this word: RZIEUSE

7. Name two reasons why people sometimes try to persuade friends to use.

8. Name two examples of drug use behavior you think are appropriate.

9. Give an example of how you would respond to a friend's request that you use a psychoactive substance when you did not want to.

10. Unscramble this word: OCALHLO

11. Name two examples of substance abuse behaviors.

12. Scenario: You are 16 years old and at a party with about ten other people. You have been dating this boy or girl for two months and he/she has never used any psychoactive drugs. Tonight, he/she has been drinking wine and smoking marijuana. He/she is getting very high. What do you do?

13. True or False: Psychoactive substances sometimes help people solve problems.

14. True or False: A strong cup of coffee will sober a person up after they have become high from using psychoactive substances.

15. True or False: If using psychoactive substances one time does not cause one to avoid problems or hurt others or him/herself, it is probably OK.

16. Unscramble this word: DCOITDIAN

17. True or False: Marijuana is not addictive.

18. True or False: A person cannot become addicted to prescription drugs.

19. True or False: People sometimes use psychoactive substances to feel part of a group.

20. Scenario: Your best friend is visiting. You have just seen him or her take a bottle from your parents' medicine cabinet. What do you do?

ANSWERS TO TEAM WORKSHEET IV

1. True

2. Addiction can develop, can lead to injuries or death, can be legally punished, judgment becomes impaired

3. False

4. Cocaine

5. True

6. Seizure

7. To dare someone, do not want to use alone, see the effects on someone else, to make a fool of someone

8. When prescribed by physician, when taken as directed, while hospitalized and given by medical staff

9. No right or wrong answer

10. Alcohol

11. Slurred speech, irrational thinking, staggering, hallucinations, hyperactivity, drowsiness

12. No right or wrong answer

13. False

14. False

15. False

16. Addiction

17. False–can produce psychological addiction

18. False

19. True

20. No right or wrong answer

WEEK IV
DAY 5
TOURNAMENT

Focus: Summarizing, integrating week's activities
Method: Game
Time: 1 period
Capsule Description: Students in their TGT teams compete for points by correctly answering questions based on the week's activities.

Divide the class into the tournament tables. Go over the rules of play again and the "GIGS" if students need reminding. Pass out Game D, Game D Answer Sheet, and Game Score Sheet to each team. Answer any questions. At the end of the tournament, fill out the Team Summary Sheet, Tournament Score Sheet, and publicize the results. Then devise new tournament tables according to the "bumping" procedure.

GAME D
PSYCHOACTIVE SUBSTANCE USE DECISIONS AND PEER PRESSURE

D-1   Name two behaviors that would clue you that someone has been using psychoactive substances.

D-2   True or False: People sometimes persuade friends to use psychoactive substances because they do not want to use alone.

D-3   Mary's mother lost her job and became depressed. Her doctor prescribed antidepressants. Is it okay for her to take them?

D-4   Give an example of your response to a friend's request that you use psychoactive substances when you do not want to.

D-5   True or False: American society does not sanction the use of psychoactive substances.

D-6   True or False: Addiction can be a consequence of abusing psychoactive substances.

D-7   It is okay to take medication prescribed for someone else if you have similar symptoms?

D-8   True or False: The ultimate decision to use or not use psychoactive substance resides with each person.

D-9   Name one example of psychoactive drug use behavior you think would be appropriate.

D-10   You are at a party with your date. You notice that he/she is drinking beer and smoking marijuana. You are concerned that he/she is getting high. What do you do?

D-11   True or False: If using psychoactive substances one time does not cause one to avoid problems or hurt others or him/herself, it is probably okay.

D-12   Can a strong cup of coffee sober up a person high on psychoactive substances?

D-13   True or False: Smoking marijuana will not lead to addiction, so it is okay to use.

D-14   You want to become a member of the most popular group at school. However, all members of the group use psychoactive substances. You have heard that they have some wild parties. One of the members has invited you to a party. You are scared about using drugs, but you are excited about socializing with group members. What do you do?

D-15   True or False: Psychoactive substances can help people solve problems.

D-16   Your best friend has obtained marijuana. He wants to come over and smoke at your house while your parents are out. You are afraid he might get high, and you are also afraid your parents might find out. How do you tell him no?

D-17   True or False: People often make decisions about drug use based on how their parents and their friends regard drug use.

D-18   True or False: A person cannot become addicted to prescription drugs.

D-19   I was the only person at a party on Saturday night who did not try crack. Now, everyone is calling me chicken. I feel angry, and I know that I was right not to use. How do I respond to the name calling?

D-20   True or False: People sometimes use psychoactive substances to feel part of a group.

GAME D ANSWER SHEET
PSYCHOACTIVE SUBSTANCE USE DECISIONS
AND PEER PRESSURE

D-1   Slurred speech, hyperactivity, distortions in reality, staggering, drowsiness, irrational thinking.

D-2   True

D-3   The antidepressants may help initially, but they would not solve the problem of unemployment.

D-4   Answers approved by class are acceptable

D-5   False

D-6   True

D-7   No

D-8   True

D-9   Sample answers given in practice session

D-10 Answers approved by class are acceptable

D-11 False

D-12 No

D-13 False

D-14   Answers approved by class are acceptable
D-15   False
D-16   Answers approved by class are acceptable
D-17   True
D-18   False
D-19   Answers approved by class are acceptable
D-20   True

WEEK V
DAY 1
ACTIVITY 15:
PSYCHOACTIVE SUBSTANCE USE AND DRIVING

Focus: Substance use and driving
Method: Questionnaire/Discussion
Time: 1 period
Capsule Description: Students answer questions about psychoactive substance use and driving and discuss the answers.

Break the class into pairs. Have the pairs complete the questionnaire at the end of this activity. Tell them not to write their names on their papers. Tabulate the results on the blackboard and then provide the correct answers, with explanations. Conclude the activity by asking the class to discuss ways in which psychoactive substance use may impair their driving ability, such as the following:

- performing normal driving tasks more slowly, including braking, turning, signaling, stopping
- passing on curves and hills
- weaving
- driving too slow or fast
- running through stop signs and stop lights
- late responses to unexpected occurrences, such as children running into the road or curves
- crossing the double line and driving out of the lane

1. Research shows that motor skills and reaction times are reduced by what percent after smoking one marijuana cigarette?
   A. 10 percent   B. 21 percent   C. 41 percent   D. 64 percent

2. While using stimulants, drivers tend to _____ when at the wheel.
   A. be more alert   B. overreact   C. fall asleep   D. no effect

3. What percentage of fatal traffic accidents involved someone who was drinking?
   A. 19 percent   B. 10 percent   C. 50 percent   D. no one knows

4. Which of the following are impaired when a driver is using depressants?
   A. vision   B. coordination   C. hearing   D. reaction time

5. What percentage of marijuana users drive while high?
   A. 8 percent   B. 30 percent   C. 70 percent   D. unknown

6. Teenagers make up 22 percent of all drivers and they make up _____ percent of the accidents involving alcohol.
   A. 44 percent   B. 10 percent   C. 71 percent   D. 24 percent

7. True or False: Hallucinogen use is especially dangerous while driving because the user's total concept of reality has and will be altered.

8. In most states a 150 lb. person is presumed to be under the influence of alcohol when he or she has had how many beers, glasses of wine, or average mixed drinks with hard liquor in two hours?
   A. 4   B. 6   C. 1-2   D. 5

9. True or False: Marijuana impairs not only central vision, but peripheral sight as well.

10. _____ is the only cure for intoxication.
    A. a cold shower   B. aspirin   C. time   D. coffee

11. Two-thirds of high school students use alcohol and drugs with regular frequency; of these, _____ percent use drugs and alcohol at least three times weekly.
    A. 15 percent   B. 85 percent   C. 33 percent   D. 50 percent

ANSWERS TO QUESTIONNAIRE

1. C–41 percent	5. C–70 percent	9. True
2. B–overreact	6. A–44 percent	10. C–time
3. C–50 percent	7. True	11. B–85 percent
4. A, B, and D	8. C–1 to 2	

WEEK V
DAY 2
ACTIVITY 16:
RESPONSIBILITY FOR OTHERS'
SUBSTANCE USE BEHAVIOR

Focus: Interpersonal responsibilities, values clarification
Method: Discussion
Time: 1 period
Capsule Description: Students engage in small group discussion revolving around issues of responsibility for other people's using behavior.

At the end of this activity are scenarios that you can use as departure points for discussing what a person's responsibilities are or should be toward people who may be abusing psychoactive substances. Have the class break into small groups and discuss each scenario, arriving at a consensus solution to the problem. You may want to ask the groups to focus their discussions on such issues as:

1. In the scenario, does the individual have a responsibility to the person who is abusing? Why or why not? If so, what is his or her responsibility to the abuser?

2. In each scenario, what alternative action should the person exercising responsibility take with regard to the abuser? Where does the responsible person's responsibility stop–how many attempts and what kind of attempts to help the abuser should he or she engage in before deciding to stop trying? Should he or she even stop trying? Why or why not?

3. What makes some people reluctant to exercise responsibility for other people who abuse psychoactive substances? Can anything be done to encourage greater responsibility? Should something be done? Why or why not?

4. In the instances in which we do not take responsibility for someone else who is abusing and something bad happens (for example, he or she drives home high and gets into an accident), are we to blame for what happens?

5. Should a host be legally responsible if he or she allows a guest to abuse psychoactive substances and the guest injures someone driving home?

When groups have completed the task, have them present their solutions and open the floor for class discussion. You may find that the specific issues bloom into a more global issue of whether we have a responsibility in general to other people who engage in self-destructive behavior or behavior that can endanger others. This value clarification is very important and useful.

Sample Scenario

1. You are 21 years old. Your best friend is 18 and wants you to buy a case of beer for his 15-year-old younger brother who plans to go drinking in the park with some friends. Will you buy it? Why or why not?

2. You were prescribed pain medication for your broken ankle. A friend stops by to visit and asks if the doctor gave you medication. When you answer yes, the friend asks if he or she could have a few. Will you give the pills to your friend? Why or why not?

3. You are host of a party after a football game. You have observed two of your friends drinking wine excessively and smoking marijuana. As they are getting ready to leave and drive home, you notice that they are very unsteady. What should you do, if anything? Why?

4. A 22-year-old man is accused of providing his 17-year-old girlfriend with liquor and cocaine. The girlfriend became high on these substances and fell in a lake and drowned. The man was engaged to his girlfriend and loved her very much. You are the judge in the case. What do you do?

5. Your best friend has been using speed. He is hyperactive and not thinking clearly. Your friend asks if he can borrow your car to go see his girlfriend with whom he has had an argument. You want to say no, but you are afraid you will make him angry. What should you say?

WEEK V
DAY 3
ACTIVITY 17:
SUBSTANCE USE AND DRIVING

Focus: Substance use and driving
Method: Story Completion/Discussion
Time: 1/2 period
Capsule Description: Students complete a story involving substance abuse and driving. Students discuss how they can tell if someone is too impaired to drive safely.

Have your students write endings to the story provided at the end of the activity. Then break the class into small groups and instruct the groups to read the completions written by other members of the group. Instruct the groups to try to agree on how people can tell if someone has used too much chemical substance to drive safely.

When the groups have completed their work, have a reporter from each group explain its conclusions to the class and list its signs of impairment on the blackboard.
For example:

- sleepiness, yawning
- slurred speech
- unstable walk
- unusual clumsiness
- distortions in thinking
- misperceptions of reality

- impatience, impulsiveness
- silly behavior
- boasting
- more sexual aggressiveness
- violence, more aggressiveness than usual

Conclude the activity by pointing out four major problems involved in identifying people who are too impaired to drive:

1. Many substance users who are impaired seem relatively sober to others in terms of how they walk, talk, or even drive. A person may claim to drive "better after drinking or using drugs than when sober because I am extra careful." However, while such abusers may have learned to compensate for some of the chemical substance's effects, an emergency situation such as a flat tire or pedestrian suddenly appearing would leave them unable to react quickly.

2. The more people use psychoactive substances, the less capable they are to judge whether they themselves are too impaired to drive.

Many people who have had several drinks or have used marijuana or stimulants really believe and feel they are perfectly capable of driving safely. A solution to this problem is to accept the opinion of a trusted friend on whether he or she is too impaired to drive.

3. A driver's underlying attitudes toward driving can become unexpectedly more pronounced after drinking too much or using other chemical substances. Some drivers become more cautious, others more reckless.

4. Marijuana adds to the alcohol effect. Drinking too much alcohol can lead to nausea and vomiting. Marijuana suppresses the "vomit center" of the brain, therefore a person can drink more than the body would normally allow, leading to higher levels of intoxication. Behind the wheel of a car and independent of each other, each is dangerous. Together, they can be fatal.

Story Beginning

This is the beginning of our story. Write an ending for it. There is no "right" answer. There are lots of ways it could end. Be as creative as you like.

The party had been going full blast for over four hours. Everyone had been having a good time–talking, joking. A lot of people had been drinking the fantastic rum punch, but there was also beer and hard liquor. Some of the people had been passing around joints of marijuana. Richard and his girlfriend, Susan, and Darrel and his girlfriend, Amy, had come to the party together and spent most of the evening talking to each other.

Richard was having an especially good time. He had been drinking beer all night and smoking some marijuana. Susan was getting a little nervous because after the last party they attended, Richard had gotten high and had too much to drink. When he drove her home he wandered over the center line and ran through a red light. So Susan decided to check on Richard during this party to see if he could drive. But it is difficult at a party to have a good time and also keep track of how much your boyfriend is drinking and/or using. Susan had spotted several clear signs that Richard was too impaired to drive, and she had talked to Paula in the ladies' room about Richard. Paula, in fact, agreed to stick up for her if she needed help in persuading Richard not to drive, because Paula had also noticed some signs that Richard should not be driving. About an hour later, Darrel suggested they all go home. But as Richard pulled out the keys to his car, Susan took him aside and said:

Write an ending for the story.

WEEK V
DAY 3
ACTIVITY 18:
SUBSTANCE USE, DRIVING, AND THE LAW

Focus: Legal aspects of substance use and driving
Method: Small Group Discussions
Time: 1 period
Capsule Description: Students engage in small group discussions about the legal consequences of substance abuse and driving. This activity consists of one initial exercise and several possible follow-up exercises.

Ask your students to divide into groups of four. Give each group one of the following scenarios about people arrested for DUI. Make sure that each scenario goes to at least two groups. Ask each group to discuss the case from the point of view of the judge who will take action (or perhaps not take action) on the case and to reach a consensus on what the action will be. After 15 minutes or so, ask a group reporter to read the group's case and report on its decision. Each reporter will also give the rationale for the group's decision for comparison and discussion.

1. Marci is a 16-year-old cheerleader from a respectable family. During her first home football game, her boyfriend, a senior, kept offering Marci sips of a soft drink to which he added rum. By the end of the game, Marci was giggly and a little unsteady on her feet but decided to drive her boyfriend to a party in her car. On the way, she was arrested for DUI.

2. Melvin is a middle-aged divorcee. He often has a drink after work and frequently goes bar-hopping. Melvin occasionally snorts cocaine. Since his own car was in the shop, Melvin had borrowed a car from a buddy. On the way to return the car to its owner, Melvin drove down the middle of the street and was arrested for DUI and

possession of cocaine. As it turned out, Melvin did not have a driver's license because it had been suspended earlier in the year.

3. John, a college student, was arrested for DUI following a football game during which his team won the national championship. He had already been arrested earlier in the year on the same charges.

4. Dave, a junior in high school, is well liked by both students and teachers. He is a passenger in a car in which the driver, a friend, has had a couple of beers and joints of marijuana. When the friend sees the blue light behind them, he pulls over on the side of the road and changes places with Dave. Dave is arrested for DUI and possession of marijuana.

As a follow-up to this activity, or as a substitute for it, your students can engage in one of the following exercises:

1. Students interview police officers about how they handle public drunkenness and other offenses such as possession of drugs and drunk driving. The scenarios which the students discussed in small groups could form the basis for the discussion. Other questions the students might ask are as follows:

- What are the laws about substance abuse and driving?
- In what kinds of situations do you usually find people driving impaired?
- What kinds of substance abuse offenses do juveniles commit?
- How do you handle them?
- What happens to them?
- What are the penalties for illegal substance abuse and driving?

2. Students evaluate possible solutions to the problem of substance abuse and driving in their community. Begin the activity by asking students to brainstorm about every idea they think would cut down on impaired driving, no matter how far-fetched the idea might be. Then ask for comments on how many of the ideas might really work, and what would have to be done to put them into operation. Sample ideas might be as follows:

- Publish names of people arrested for DUI in the newspaper.
- Take a person's license away on the first offense.
- Legislate a two-drink limit at every bar.

WEEK V
DAY 4
TEAM PRACTICE SESSION

Focus: Preparations for TGT tournament
Method: Worksheets
Time: 1 period
Capsule Description: The students work in their TGT teams on specially prepared worksheets in preparation for the TGT tournament.

Divide the class members into their TGT teams and let them complete the worksheets in their small groups. Instruct the class to discuss each question, coming to a consensus answer for each question. Circulate throughout the class to check the groups' progress and answer any questions. When all groups are finished with worksheets, go over them with correct answers so that if they like they may study for the tournament tomorrow.

TEAM WORKSHEET V

1. After how many arrests for DUI in your state does a person become a "habitual offender" and lose his/her license?

2. True or False: While using stimulants, drivers tend to overreact when at the wheel.

3. Name two options you would have if your boyfriend/girlfriend got too drunk to drive you home from a party but you had to get home by your curfew at 11:00 p.m.

4. In most states a 150 lb. person is presumed to be under the influence when he or she has had how many beers, glasses of wine, or average mixed drinks in two hours?

5. True or False: When a person becomes high and drives, it is human nature that the person will become more cautious than normal.

6. _____ is the only cure for intoxication.

7. Name one reason why some people would be reluctant to exercise responsibility for other people who abuse psychoactive substances.

8. True or False: When a driver has used depressants, his/her vision, coordination, and reaction time become impaired.

9. Name two signs that would clue you that a person is too high to drive.

10. True or False: A person should never admit to a girlfriend/boyfriend that she/he cannot drive because of substance abuse–it is more important to be able to "hold your liquor."

11. True or False: Research shows that motor skills and reaction times are reduced by 41 percent after smoking one marijuana cigarette.

12. True or False: 50 percent of fatal traffic accidents involve someone who was drinking.

13. A person 16 years old or younger arrested for DUI would:
    A. be on probation until he/she turned 18
    B. be released to his/her parents
    C. be adjudicated in juvenile court
    D. be suspended from school

14. Passing on curves and hills and weaving are two ways a drunk person might drive that are different from most sober drivers.

15. True or False: 70 percent of marijuana users drive while high.

16. True or False: It is not especially dangerous to use hallucinogens while driving.

17. Name one reason why a host should be declared legally responsible if a person abuses chemical substances at her/his party and later that person injures someone in a car accident.

18. The _____ people drink, the _____ capable they are of judging whether they are too drunk to drive.

19. True or False: More than 60 percent of all motor vehicle fatalities are alcohol and drug related.

ANSWERS TO TEAM WORKSHEET V

1. Instructor obtain answer for individual state.

2. True

3. Get someone else to drive, ride a bus, call parents, etc.

4. 1-2

5. False

6. Time

7. Afraid of person's reaction, not wanting to get involved, etc.

8. True

9. Slurred speech, slower movements, sleepiness, silly behavior, lack of concentration, etc.

10. False

11. True

12. True

13. C

14. True

15. True

16. False

17. The host is responsible for the party and should stop others from over-using or not using or find them other ways to get home.

18. More, less

19. True

WEEK V
DAY 5
TOURNAMENT

Focus: Summarizing, integrating week's activities
Method: Game
Time: 1 period
Capsule Description: Students in their TGT teams compete for points by correctly answering questions based on the week's activities.

Divide the class into the tournament tables. Go over the rules of play again and the "GIGS" if students need reminding. Pass out Game E, Game E Answer Sheet, and Game Score Sheet to each team. Answer any questions. At the end of the tournament, fill out the Team Summary Sheet, Tournament Score Sheet, and publicize the results. Then devise new tournament tables according to the "bumping" procedure.

GAME E
PSYCHOACTIVE SUBSTANCE USE AND DRIVING

E-1   Why would it be dangerous to drive after taking depressants?

E-2   In most states a 150 lb. person is presumed to be under the influence when he or she has had how many beers, glasses of wine, or average mixed drinks in two hours?

E-3   True or False: 70 percent of all marijuana users drive while high.

E-4   What would happen to a person 16 years or younger arrested for DUI?

E-5   Should a host be held legally responsible if someone abuses chemical substances at her/his party and later injures someone in a car accident?

E-6   After how many arrests for DUI in your state does a person become an habitual offender and lose his/her license?

E-7   True or False: It is okay to use stimulants and drive.

E-8   What percentage of fatal accidents involved someone who was intoxicated?

E-9   True or False: Teenagers make up 44 percent of the accidents involving alcohol.

E-10   Your date has taken LSD. You are afraid to ride home from the party with him/her. What do you do?

E-11   True or False: A person should never admit to a girlfriend/boyfriend that she/he cannot drive because of substance use–it is more important to be able to "hold your liquor."

E-12   True or False: Research shows that motor skills and reaction time are reduced by 41 percent after smoking one marijuana cigarette.

E-13   What is the only cure for intoxication?

E-14   Are people more cautious than normal after becoming high and then driving?

E-15   Why is driving especially dangerous after hallucinogen use?

E-16   True or False: More than 60 percent of all motor vehicle fatalities are alcohol and drug-related.

E-17   True or False: Marijuana impairs only a user's central vision, not peripheral vision.

E-18   True or False: The more people use psychoactive substances, the less capable they are to judge whether they themselves are too impaired to drive.

E-19   A friend, using cocaine, has become upset with his girlfriend. He wants to borrow your car to go find her and talk. You do not want to lend him your car, but you are afraid he will get mad if you say no. What do you do?

E-20   Name one reason why a person should take responsibility for helping a substance abuser.

E-21   Would a person under the influence of chemical substances likely be able to avoid hitting a pedestrian who suddenly stepped in the road? Why or why not?

GAME E ANSWER SHEET
PSYCHOACTIVE SUBSTANCE USE AND DRIVING

E-1   Vision, coordination, and reaction time become impaired

E-2   1-2

E-3   True

E-4   He/she would be adjudicated in juvenile court

E-5   Answers approved by class are acceptable

E-6   Instructor supply answer

E-7   False

E-8   50 percent

E-9   True

E-10   Examples: Try to get him/her to let you drive; try to get another ride; call a taxi; call parents to come get you.

E-11   False

E-12   True

E-13   Time

E-14   No

E-15   The user's total concept of reality has and will be altered

E-16   True

E-17   False

E-18   True

E-19   Answers approved by class are acceptable

E-20   To keep the person from hurting him/herself while impaired.

E-21   No–the person would not be able to react appropriately.

WEEK VI
DAY 1
ACTIVITY 19:
PSYCHOACTIVE SUBSTANCE USE AND DEPENDENCE

Focus: Chemical dependence
Method: Questionnaire, discussion, mini-lecture
Time: 1 period
Capsule Description: Students explore their conceptions about addiction and correct any misconceptions they have.

The activity has three parts. You may use one, two, or all three parts, but if you choose to use all, it is best to use them in the order provided.

1. Distribute copies of the chemical dependence questionnaire provided at the end of this activity, or read the questions aloud and have the students record their answers on note paper. Tabulate the results of the class on the blackboard. If you plan to use the second part of this activity, present the correct answers later after that exercise. If several students incorrectly answered a particular question, explore with the class why misconceptions of people who are dependent on psychoactive substance might be so prevalent. See if the class can identify any additional misconceptions the public may have about chemical dependence.

2. Write the phrase "chemical dependence" on the blackboard. Ask your students to jot down on a piece of paper (or brainstorm orally) all the words or phrases that come to mind when they hear or see the phrase "chemical dependence." Have your students determine, as best they can, if the class has an accurate conception about the nature of chemical dependence. The need for corrective information can be met by the third part of this exercise.

3. Present as much information about chemical dependence as you deem appropriate to the needs of your students. Provided below are some outlined topics you might want to cover.

1. The Person Dependent on Psychoactive Substances

On the simplest level, the substance abuser is anyone for whom the use of psychoactive substances creates a problem. Example: psychological–judgment is impaired; social–person says or does aggressive things he/she would not normally do; financial–person spends more on psychoactive substance than he/she can afford. The people dependent on psychoactive substances are individuals who once they begin using cannot normally predict or control how much or how long they will use. Example: a person dependent on cocaine will continuously use the drug until the supply is exhausted.

2. Early Signs of Chemical Dependence

- Drinks/uses to calm nerves
- Lying about how often and how much consumed
- Preoccupation with alcohol/drugs

- Showing marked personality changes when drinking/using
- Becoming neglectful of health

Chemical dependence is a chronic, progressive, potentially fatal disease. It is characterized by tolerance, physical and/or psychological dependency, or dangerous changes to body organs.

- Chronic and progressive indicate that the physical, social and/or emotional changes are cumulative and get worse if the person continues to drink/use.
- Tolerance–the brain has adapted to the presence of high concentrations of the chemical substance. As a result, more of the substance is needed to achieve the same high as before.
- Physical dependency–there are withdrawal symptoms upon decreasing or ceasing consumption of the chemical substance (examples of withdrawal signs are shakiness, fast pulse rate, increased blood pressure, nausea, sweatiness, having delirium tremens, in extreme cases).
- Psychological dependency–people depend on the chemical substance to make them feel better. People who are psychologically dependent become aware of dependency when they can not get the drug they are used to. They feel rotten. All they can think of is getting more of the chemical substance.

3. Typical Person with Chemical Dependence

People who abuse and/or are dependent on psychoactive substances come from all walks of life–all races, socioeconomic levels, employment levels, lifestyles. The stereotype of the skid row bum as a portrayal of all persons dependent on chemical substances is a myth.

4. Chemical Dependence–Theories of Causation

There are different theories on what causes chemical dependence. Certain researchers think physiology is the cause–that those persons dependent on psychoactive substances lack a certain enzyme or have a genetic abnormality that makes them vulnerable to chemical dependence. Another theory is that the use of psychoactive substance is learned behavior, and those who do not learn to use it properly develop problems. A third theory is that because society accepts the use of medication to alleviate psychological, physical, or emotional pain, chemical dependence exists. Finally, a fourth theory is that chemical dependence is caused by psychological difficulties, such as having a low tolerance for frustration, using chemical substances when depressed to alleviate bad feelings, and being self-destructive by using chemical substances to harm oneself.

CHEMICAL DEPENDENCE QUESTIONNAIRE

Myth or Fact?

_____ 1. A person dependent on psychoactive substances is someone who usually cannot stop drinking or using once he/she ingests the substance.

_____ 2. It is impossible for someone to become chemically dependent by using/drinking just once.

_____ 3. All psychoactive substances have the potential for dependence.

_____ 4. Almost all people who are dependent on pyschoactive substances are men.

_____ 5. Most people who are chemically dependent have jobs and live with their families.

_____ 6. Psychoactive substance abusers are often chemically dependent persons in an early stage of their disease.

_____ 7. Once people become chemically dependent, it is too late to help them.

_____ 8. Psychoactive substance abusers can sometimes control how often and how much they drink/use; persons dependent on chemical substances usually cannot.

_____ 9. Someone can be physically dependent and/or psychologically dependent on psychoactive substances.

_____10. A person can be dependent on a chemical substance without experiencing psychological withdrawal symptoms upon cessation of the substance.

ANSWERS TO QUESTIONNAIRE

1. Fact	4. Fact	7. Myth	10. Fact
2. Myth	5. Fact	8. Fact	
3. Fact	6. Fact	9. Fact	

WEEK VI
DAY 2
ACTIVITY 20
EXPLORING ATTITUDES TOWARD PSYCHOACTIVE SUBSTANCE USE AND DEPENDENCE

Focus: Attitudes toward chemical dependence
Method: Writing/discussion/role play
Time: 1 period
Capsule Description: Students describe how they might respond to a problem abuser in the family and/or role play scenes in which a parent is concerned about his/her child's friendship with the child of a chemically dependent person and then discuss the attitudes toward chemical dependence revealed in the simulation.

This activity has two options which may be used consecutively or alone.

Option 1

Have students write responses to one or more of the "Dear Abby" letters provided at the end of the activity. Then break the class into small groups and instruct them to read all the responses of their members, discuss the best response–and write down this new, improved response. Have each group present its response to the rest of the class and compare the results. Be sure the groups explain why they feel their response is a good one and will help the person who wrote in.

Conduct a follow-up discussion that focuses on:

- the various options that family members can choose to cope with psychoactive substance abuse.
- attitudes (such as stereotyping) and feeling (ex: disgust, pity, fear, anger) expressed in the letters or the responses toward substance abuse families and substance abusing.

Option 2

Group the students into pairs and give each student in each pair a role profile (child or parent) from among those supplied at the end of the activity or ones developed by you. Have each pair of students role play its scenario by itself. Circulate around the room, listening in on the various conversations, stimulating discussion where necessary.

Have several pairs present their solutions or cause for the deadlock to the class, and have one or two volunteers reenact their role plays for the class.

Lead discussion on the following:

- how did the student feel about the chemically dependent persons he/she portrayed in his/her parts?
- what attitudes toward chemical dependence were revealed in the role plays?
- which of the attitudes expressed were appropriate? inappropriate? why?

Option 1: Sample "Dear Abby" Letters

How Will You Respond?

Dear Abby,

My husband plays poker with a group of his male friends once a week. About a month ago, one of his friends brought some cocaine the night they played. My husband and a few others tried cocaine. Since then every time they play, they use cocaine. My husband got really high last week and wasn't able to go to sleep when he got home. I am worried. What can I do?

Concerned

*   *   *

How Will You Respond?

Dear Abby,

My father frequently goes on drinking sprees, some of which last for several days. When he is not drinking, he is kind and fun. But when he drinks too much he is mean, sloppy, and sometimes violent. What can I do? I am 14 years old.

Concerned

*   *   *

How Will You Respond?

Dear Abby,

My mother spends all day watching soap operas or sleeping. My father works two jobs because we have a big family, so he is not home much. My mom takes some kind of pills for her nerves and sometimes she acts groggy and slurs her words. When I get home from school, she makes me clean the house and cook dinner. When I want to be with friends or listen to music, she gets really mad. What can I do?

Trapped

*   *   *

Option 2: Sample Roles for Role Play

Parent:

Whenever you pick up your son from little league practice or games, you see him talking with Richard Smith, another player. The few times you have come early, you have noticed that they sit together on the bench and talk when not playing.

Richard's father, Joe Smith, has been in treatment at least twice for substance abuse. One of the guys at the office lives next door to the Smiths and has told you that Joe has been acting high lately and that Joe and his wife have been having loud arguments. You have never met Richard, but you know that one of his two brothers has been arrested for possession of marijuana.

You are afraid your son will get some bad ideas from Richard, and he never tells you what they talk about even though you have asked. You do not like their friendship and do not want it to become more serious.

It is dinnertime now and you are at the table with your son. You decide now is the time to raise the subject. What do you say?

Son:

While playing little league baseball, you have become friendly with Richard Smith. He is a good ball player and tells funny stories about some of the wild parties he hears about from his older brothers.

You know from gossip that Richard's father has been involved in drug use, and Richard has told you–he tries to hide nothing. But because Richard's father has been dependent on chemical substances, it makes Richard seem a little more interesting to you, since your father is a very quiet man. You wonder what it is like to have a father that gets high and boisterous.

Yesterday during the game, Richard told you his father was going to take him to the Boston Red Sox game on Sunday and invited you to join them. You do not usually get a chance to go to a big league game and you really want to go. Secretly, you are also very curious to meet Richard's father.

It is dinner time now at your house and you figure you had better tell your parents where you are going on Sunday. You wonder if they will object. What do you say?

WEEK VI
DAY 3
ACTIVITY 21:
TREATMENT FOR CHEMICAL DEPENDENCE

Focus: Treatment approaches to chemical dependence
Method: Interviews/small group/class discussion
Time: 1 period plus time outside of class
Capsule Description: Students interview local community "experts" in the field of chemical dependence treatment and then decide how they would spend funds devoted to chemical dependence treatment.

This activity has two sections–the first one must be completed outside of class and the second takes place within the classroom period.

Part I:

Divide your class into small groups and have the students within each group choose partners. Assign each group a type of local "expert" to interview. Each pair of students within one group will interview a similar expert. Examples of community experts involved in the treatment of chemical dependence are social workers and psychologists in mental health, workers on telephone hotlines, physicians, nurses, guidance counselors at schools, public and mental health officials.

Instruct the students to ask for information about treatment for substance abusers/dependence–what is available in the community, what particular type of treatment each expert favors. Have the students take notes during the interview as they will need information for Part II of this activity.

Part II:

During the regularly scheduled class meeting have the students gather in their small groups with their interview notes handy. Present them with the following scenario and ask them to reach a group consensus on how to best deal with the problem, sharing the information they learned doing the interviews in Part I.

Scenario: The federal government is prepared to give your state

$200,000 for whatever project(s) you choose that will either prevent substance abuse problems, treat existing substance abuse problems, or both. The one condition the government has made is that the entire class must agree on what the money will be spent on–what the projects will be. The small groups will be given half the period to decide how they think the money should be spent. Then each group will present its solution, explaining the rationale behind it. The entire class will discuss all proposals and, hopefully, come to a unified decision. If by the end of the class period, the class cannot decide how the money should be spent, the state will lose the money.

You may want to center the class discussion around some of the following points:

1. Should more emphasis be placed on preventing psychoactive substance abuse or treating it?

2. Which prevention approaches are likely to be the most effective and why? Which treatment approaches are likely to help the greatest number of substance abusers and why?

3. Did the group tend to compete rather than cooperate? Why? Is this what happens in society at large? Who competes for funds devoted to preventing and treating substance abuse?

4. Was cooperation high within each group but low between groups or vice versa?

5. Did the group generate several ideas before selecting one or did they begin with a single idea that went uncontested? Why? Did everyone in each group agree to the decisions made? How were decisions made? Is this what happens in society at large?

WEEK VI
DAY 4
TEAM PRACTICE SESSION

Focus: Preparation for TGT tournament
Method: Worksheets
Time: 1 period
Capsule Description: The students work in their TGT teams on specially prepared worksheets in preparation for the TGT tournament.

Divide the class members into their TGT teams and let them work the worksheets in these small groups. Instruct the class to discuss each question as a group, coming to a consensus answer for each question. Circulate throughout the class to check the groups' progress and answer any questions. When all groups are finished with the worksheets, go over them as a class and provide them with correct answers so that they may study if they like for the tournament tomorrow.

TEAM WORKSHEET VI

1. Name one symptom of chemical dependence that occurs in the early phase.

2. On the simplest level, the problem drinker or user is anyone for whom the use of a chemical substance _____ _____ _____.

3. True or False: If a chemically dependent person really wanted to, he/she could stop drinking/using to excess.

4. True or False: Chemically dependent people are inferior to everyone else because they drink/use too much.

5. What does progressive mean?

6. If a person has a substance abuse problem and continues to drink/use, one could expect the physical, social or emotional changes in the person to get better or worse?

7. True or False: Tolerance means the brain has adapted to the high concentration of chemical substance (used) in the body, and so it takes less to achieve the same high as before.

8. True or False: Physical dependency means that a person would get withdrawal symptoms upon decreasing or ceasing the use of the chemical substance.

9. True or False: In comparing chemical dependence with other illnesses in terms of the seriousness of its consequences, chemical dependence would rank high.

10. True or False: Society is very unified about the cause of psychoactive substance abuse/dependence.

11. Name two different theories about what causes chemical dependence.

12. Name the groups that meet to support alcohol dependents and drug dependents in their decision to abstain from drinking/using.

13. True or False: Chemical dependency is a public health problem because the victims of abuse/dependency cannot cope with their condition themselves.

14. Is there a typical person who is chemically dependent? Why or why not?

15. Would you say a depressed person who frequently drinks to feel better is on the way to developing a problem with drinking? Why or why not?

16. Which of the following is not accepted as a possible cause of chemical dependence?
    A. nutritional deficiency   C. a genetic deficiency
    B. personality factors   D. a learned behavior

17. In the later stages of chemical dependence, the person often has all but which characteristic?
    A. a system of alibis about why he/she drinks/uses
    B. a lack of faith in religion
    C. an accepted belief that no one cares about him/her
    D. a loss of self-respect

18. True or False: Most chemically dependent people are men.

19. True or False: Most communities have counselors available who are trained to help chemically dependent persons with their problems.

20. True or False: It is important for family members of a chemically dependent person to talk to someone about how chemical dependency has affected their life.

21. Name two resources a family would have in the community to help deal with problems as a result of a family member's chemical dependency.

ANSWERS TO TEAM WORKSHEET VI

1. Drinking/using to calm nerves or because of unhappiness; lying about how often and/or how much consumed; preoccupation with alcohol/drugs; showing marked personality changes when drinking or using; becoming neglectful of health

2. Causes a problem

3. False

4. False

5. The changes are cumulative and get worse if a person continues to drink/use

6. Worse

7. False

8. True

9. True

10. False

11. Physiology–a genetic abnormality; a destructive learned behavior; society's acceptance of psychoactive substance use; psychological difficulties

12. Alcoholics Anonymous, Narcotics Anonymous, Cocaine Anonymous

13. True

14. No–chemically dependent people come from all walks of life–socioeconomic status, race, religion

15. Yes–the person is coping with problems by using alcohol

16. A

17. B

18. False

19. True

20. True

21. AA, NA, CA mental health professionals, public health professionals, guidance counselors, clergy

WEEK VI
DAY 5
TOURNAMENT

Focus: Summarizing, integrating week's activities
Method: Game
Time: 1 period
Capsule Description: Students in their TGT teams compete for points by correctly answering questions based on the week's activities.

Divide the class into the tournament tables. Go over the rules of play again and the "GIGS" if students need reminding. Pass out Game F, Game F Answer Sheet, and Game Score Sheet to each team. Answer any questions. At the end of the tournament, fill out the Team Summary Sheet, Tournament Score Sheet, and publicize the results. Then devise new tournament tables according to the "bumping" procedure.

GAME F
PSYCHOACTIVE SUBSTANCE USE
AND DEPENDENCE

F-1   Could a chemically dependent person stop drinking or using to excess if he/she really wanted to?

F-2   True or False: Progressive means that changes in substance use are cumulative and get worse if a person continues to drink or use.

F-3   Would you say a depressed person who frequently drinks to feel better is on the way to developing a problem with drinking? Why or why not?

F-4   True or False: Physical dependency means that a person would get withdrawal symptoms upon decreasing or ceasing the use of the chemical substance.

F-5   Is genetic abnormality considered to be one theory regarding the cause of chemical dependency?

F-6   True or False: Chemical dependency is not regarded as a public health problem.

F-7   True or False: Most chemically dependent people are men.

F-8   Would AA be a good resource to help a person who is chemically dependent?

F-9   True or False: It is important for family members of a chemically dependent person to talk with someone about how chemical dependency has affected his/her life.

F-10 On the simplest level, the problem drinker or user is anyone for whom the use of a chemical substance _____ _____ _____ .

F-11 True or False: Chemically dependent people are inferior to everyone else because they drink/use too much.

F-12 If a person has a substance abuse problem and continues to drink or use, could one expect the physical, social, or emotional changes in the person to get better or worse?

F-13   True or False: Lying about how often and/or how much is consumed is one symptom of chemical dependence that occurs in the early phase.

F-14   True or False: In comparing chemical dependence with other illnesses in terms of the seriousness of its consequence, chemical dependence would rank high.

F-15   True or False: Tolerance means the brain has adapted to the high concentrations of the chemical substance (used) in the body, and so it takes less to achieve the same high as before.

F-16   Is society unified about the cause of psychoactive substance abuse?

F-17   True or False: Nutritional deficiency is accepted as a cause of chemical dependency.

F-18   Is there a typical person who is chemically dependent? Why or why not?

F-19   True or False: Al-anon is a self-help group for families of chemically dependent persons.

F-20   True or False: In the later stages of chemical dependence, the person often has a system of alibis about why he/she drinks or uses.

GAME F ANSWER SHEET
PSYCHOACTIVE SUBSTANCE USE
AND DEPENDENCE

F-1   No
F-2   True
F-3   Yes–the person is coping with problems by using alcohol
F-4   True
F-5   Yes
F-6   False
F-7   False

F-8   Yes
F-9   True
F-10 Causes a problem
F-11 False
F-12 Worse
F-13 True
F-14 True
F-15 False
F-16 No
F-17 False
F-18 No–chemically dependent people come from all walks of life–socioeconomic status, race, religion
F-19 True
F-20 True

POSTTEST

1. Alcohol is:
   A. a stimulant
   B. an anesthetic
   C. a narcotic
   D. a sedative-hypnotic drug

2. The effects of stimulant abuse can cause:
   A. aggressive behavior
   B. panic
   C. hallucinations
   D. all of the above

3. The _____ metabolizes psychoactive substance.
   A. stomach   B. liver   C. kidneys   D. gall bladder

4. The number of deaths annually that are directly attributable to substance abuse is:
   A. 15,000 to 20,000
   B. 8,000 to 10,000
   C. 100,000 to 120,000
   D. 45,000 to 50,000

5. Cocaine is:
   A. a hallucinogen
   B. a depressant
   C. a narcotic
   D. a stimulant

6. Which of the following is not accepted as a possible cause of chemical dependence?

   A. nutritional deficiency   C. genetic deficiency
   B. personality factors   D. a learned behavior

7. Heroin is synthesized from morphine and is _____ times as potent.

   A. 3   B. 10   C. 18   D. 35

8. In the later stages of chemical dependence, the person often has all but which characteristic?

   A. a system of alibis about why he/she drinks or uses
   B. an accepted belief that no one cares about him/her
   C. a lack of faith in religion
   D. a loss of self-respect

9. The two most commonly used and abused drugs in America are:

   A. alcohol and cocaine   C. alcohol and heroin
   B. marijuana and depressants   D. alcohol and marijuana

10. Teenagers use drugs:

   A. to have a good time
   B. to be part of the group
   C. to get their minds off of problems or escape
   D. all of the above

11. _____ is the most common contaminant found in a number of street drugs.

   A. PCP   B. codeine   C. heroin   D. crack

12. Two-thirds of high school students use alcohol and drugs with regular frequency. Of these, _____ percent use drugs and alcohol at least three times weekly.

   A. 15 percent   B. 85 percent   C. 33 percent   D. 50 percent

13. _____ is the only cure for intoxication.
    A. Coffee   B. Time   C. Cold Shower   D. Carbonated drink

14. Research shows that motor skills and reaction time are reduced by _____ percent after smoking one marijuana cigarette.
    A. 5 percent   B. 17 percent   C. 41 percent   D. 25 percent

15. A form of amnesia, lasting from seconds to days, resulting from alcohol use is a:
    A. Blackout   B. Seizure   C. Convulsion   D. Delirium

16. _____ percent of all teen suicide attempts are via drug overdoses.
    A. 15 percent   B. 73 percent   C. 29 percent   D. 88 percent

True or False:

17. A user becomes tolerant to chemicals and requires more and more to get the same high.

18. A slang term for amphetamines is uppers.

19. Sniffing inhalants can lead to sudden death.

20. Only the use of narcotics leads to drug addiction.

21. Withdrawal from alcohol or other depressants can result in death.

22. Cough syrups containing codeine are classified as depressants.

23. Marijuana use has been proven to result in cellular damage to the body.

24. Depressants used in combination with alcohol are not potentially fatal.

25. The repeated use of narcotics results in increased tolerance.

26. Moderate to heavy marijuana use by males results in a decreased sperm count and an abundance of abnormally formed sperm.

27. It is okay to take medication prescribed for someone else if you have similar symptoms.

28. Marijuana can be addicting.

29. People sometimes use psychoactive substances to feel part of a group.

30. When a person becomes high and drives, it is human nature that the person will become more cautious than normal.

31. If a chemically dependent person really wanted to, he/she could stop drinking or using to excess.

32. Society is very unified about the cause of psychoactive substance abuse/dependence.

33. Most chemically dependent people are men.

34. Withdrawal from narcotics produces physical discomfort but does not result in death.

35. An overdose of cannabis can produce psychosis.

36. The media does not really influence how people view using psychoactive substances.

37. Psychoactive substances get to the bloodstream almost as soon as they are ingested.

38. More teenagers die in drug- and alcohol-related motor vehicle accidents than from any disease.

39. Physical dependency means that a person would get withdrawal symptoms upon decreasing or ceasing the use of chemical substance.

40. A person cannot become addicted to prescription drugs.

41. Once psychoactive substances enter the brain they do not circulate back through the body again.

42. Studies have shown that chronic exposure to some solvents and gasoline causes severe anemia and leukemia.

43. The effects of marijuana on female reproduction are of short duration.

44. The intravenous injection of narcotics or other substances can result in hepatitis, AIDS, or other infections from contaminated needles.

45. Two reasons why people sometimes try to persuade friends to use drugs are to see the effects on someone else or because they do not want to use alone.

46. Heavy drinking for a long period of time may cause physical problems but does not cause brain damage.

47. Dependency on crack can occur in as little as two weeks.

48. When psychoactive substances are snorted or inhaled they go directly to the brain.

49. A strong cup of coffee will sober a person up after she/he becomes high from using psychoactive substances.

50. When using stimulants, drivers tend to overreact at the wheel.

51. It is important for family members with a chemically dependent person in the family to talk to someone about how chemical dependency has affected her/his life.

52. Seventy percent of marijuana users drive while high.

53. LSD is a stimulant.

54. The effects of PCP can last for days.

POSTTEST ANSWER SHEET

1. D	21. True	41. False
2. D	22. False	42. True
3. B	23. True	43. False
4. C	24. False	44. True
5. D	25. True	45. True
6. A	26. True	46. False
7. B	27. False	47. True
8. C	28. True	48. False
9. D	29. True	49. False
10. D	30. False	50. True
11. A	31. False	51. True
12. B	32. False	52. True
13. B	33. False	53. False
14. C	34. True	54. True
15. A	35. True	
16. D	36. False	
17. True	37. True	
18. True	38. True	
19. True	39. True	
20. False	40. False	

REFERENCES

Allman, R., Taylor, H. A. & Nathan, P. E. (1972). Group drinking during stress: Effects on drinking behavior, affect and psychopathology. *American Journal of Psychiatry,* 129 (6): 45-54.

Botvin, G. J., Baker, E., Filazzola, A. D., & Botvin, E. M. (1990). A cognitive-behavioral approach to substance abuse prevention: One-year follow-up. *Addictive Behaviors,* 15, 47-63.

Botvin, G. J., & Wills, T. A. (1985). Personal and social skills training: Cognitive-behavioral approaches to substance abuse prevention. In C. Bell & R. J. Battjes (Eds.), *Prevention Research: Deterring Drug Abuse Among Children and Adolescents* (pp. 8-49) (NIDA Research Monograph No. 63). Washington, DC: U.S. Government Printing Office.

Ellickson, P. L. & Bell, R. M. (1990). Drug prevention in junior high: A multi-site longitudinal test. *Science,* 247:1299-1305.

Kandel, D. B. (1986). Processes of peer influence in adolescence. In R. Silberstein (Ed.), *Development as Action in Context: Problem Behavior and Normal Youth Development* (pp. 203-228). New York: Springer-Verlag.

Ladd, G. W. & Asher, S. R. (1985). Social skill training and children's peer relations: Current issues in research and practice. In L. L. Abate & M. A. Milan (Eds.), *Handbook of Social Skills Training and Research* (pp. 219-244). New York: Wiley.

Ramey, C. T., Bryant, D. M., Campbell, F. A., Sparling, J. J., & Wasik, B. H. (1988). Early intervention for high-risk children: The Carolina Early Intervention Program. In R. H. Price, E. L. Cowen, R. P. Lorion, & J. Ramos-McKay (Eds.), *14 Ounces of Prevention: A Casebook for Practitioners* (pp. 32-43). Washington, DC: American Psychological Association.

Chapter 4

Adolescent Substance Abuse:
The Parent Component

Data indicate that parents whose adolescents are at risk face multiple social and psychological difficulties. The clearest empirical finding with regard to adolescents at risk seems to be the lack of knowledge by the parent or parents and the consequent lack of effectiveness in managing the child's behavior in a manner that facilitates his/her psychological and social development. It has also been pointed out that another common feature of relationships between parents and adolescents at risk is unrealistic expectations by the parents regarding what is appropriate behavior for their child (Cowen & Work, 1988; Howing, Hawkins, Lishner, Catalano, & Howard, 1986; Patterson & Forgatch, 1987; Wodarski & Thyer, 1989).

Another empirical finding of note has been the high degree of strain evident in families. Family interaction patterns have been characterized as primarily negative; that is, parents engage in excessive amounts of criticism, threats, negative statements, physical punishment, and a corresponding lack of positive interaction such as positive statements, praise, positive physical contact, and so forth (Bock & English, 1973; Brandon & Folk, 1977; Brennan, Huizinga, & Elliott, 1978; Hildebrand, 1968; Robin & Foster, 1989; Robinson, 1978; Suddick, 1973; Vandeloo, 1977). In view of this finding, a comprehensive prevention approach should include appropriate interventions that teach knowledge about the problems adolescents face, substance use issues, communication skills, problem solving, and conflict resolution to family members. This chapter presents the five-week parental component of our dual intervention.

WEEK I

In this session, you will survey a gamut of topics related to drug use, such as how much of a drug a body can absorb in a given length of time, the physiological attributes of drugs in relation to the human body, the amount of alcohol in a variety of alcoholic beverages, and how to assess a drug problem.

(1) Drugs and Our Society

Adolescents comprise a unique population because they are in a state of change and confusion as their bodies develop and grow; as they begin to contemplate the future and develop goals; as they begin assessing their own feelings, ideas, and attitudes; and as they search for their own identity or sense of self. They often enter a "period of free experimentation before a final sense of identity is achieved" (Zastrow & Kirst-Ashman, 1987, p. 200). Also, because adolescence can be such a stressful and painful time in one's life, fraught with feelings of awkwardness and inadequacies, the individual will try to alleviate this pain. Whether the individual is simply experimenting or whether she/he is trying to reduce the turmoils of adolescence, drugs and/or alcohol may be a factor.

In 1982, sixty-one billion dollars were spent on alcohol and drugs in the United States. Nine out of ten tenth graders have been drunk at least once. Eighty percent of all children begin to use alcohol by seven years of age. One-third of high school students are drunk at least six times per year. There are 3.3 million teenage alcoholics in the United States today. More dollars were spent during the decade of the 1970s on alcohol than on gasoline, and taxes from this drug are the second leading source of income in this country.

Alcohol and marijuana are the two most commonly used and abused drugs. Ninety percent of high school seniors have tried marijuana and one out of thirteen are daily users. Sixty million Americans have tried marijuana and more than twenty million are regular users. Illegally grown marijuana is the fourth largest cash crop in this country. Quaaludes and cocaine are currently two of the more popularly abused substances. Cocaine use has become a status symbol and appears to be a rapidly growing democratic craze. . . . PCP [or "Angel Dust"] is illegal and manufactured only in street labs. There are many different forms or analogs of PCP, and all are extremely toxic. Dangerous abnormal reactions may occur with ingestion. PCP is the most common contaminant found in a number of other street substances. (Morrison, 1985, p. 2)

(2) What Are Drugs?

A drug is any habit-forming substance that directly affects the brain; it is a chemical substance that affects moods, perceptions, bodily functions, or consciousness and that has the potential for misuse as it may be harmful to the user (Zastrow & Kirst-Ashman, 1987, p. 221).

On the following pages is a test concerning drugs and alcohol. Please take a few minutes to answer the questions. When you have finished, we will spend some time discussing the test. Following the test are several pages of information on drugs. After the test and discussion, read over these pages. Once you have read them we will go over them.

ALCOHOL AND DRUG TEST

1. Alcohol is:
   A. a stimulant
   B. an anesthetic
   C. a narcotic
   D. a sedative-hypnotic drug

2. The effects of stimulant abuse can cause:
   A. aggressive behavior
   B. panic
   C. hallucinations
   D. all of the above

3. The _____ metabolizes psychoactive substances.
   A. stomach
   B. liver
   C. kidneys
   D. gall bladder

4. The number of deaths annually that are directly attributable to substance abuse is:
   A. 15,000 to   20,000
   B.   8,000 to   10,000
   C. 100,000 to 200,000
   D. 45,000 to   50,000

5. Cocaine is:
   A. a hallucinogen
   B. a depressant
   C. a narcotic
   D. a stimulant

6. Which of the following is not accepted as a possible cause of chemical dependency?
   A. nutritional deficiency
   B. personality factors
   C. genetic deficiency
   D. a learned behavior

7. Heroin is synthesized from morphine and is _____ times as potent.
   A. 3
   B. 10
   C. 18
   D. 35

8. In the later stages of chemical dependence, the person often has all but which characteristic?
   A. a system of alibis about why she/he drinks or uses
   B. an accepted belief that no one cares about him/her
   C. a lack of faith in religion
   D. a loss of self-respect

9. The two most commonly used and abused drugs in America are:
   A. alcohol and cocaine
   B. marijuana and depressants
   C. alcohol and heroin
   D. alcohol and marijuana

10. Teenagers use drugs:
    A. to have a good time
    B. to be part of the group
    C. to get their minds off of problems or as an escape
    D. all of the above

11. _____ is the most common contaminant found in a number of street drugs.
    A. PCP
    B. codeine
    C. heroin
    D. crack

12. Two-thirds of high school students use alcohol and drugs with regular frequency. Of these, _____ percent use drugs and alcohol at least three times weekly.
    A. 15 percent
    B. 85 percent
    C. 33 percent
    D. 50 percent

13. _____ is the only cure for intoxication.
    A. coffee
    B. time
    C. cold shower
    D. carbonated drink

14. Research shows that motor skills and reaction time are reduced by _____ percent after smoking one marijuana cigarette.
    A. 5 percent
    B. 17 percent
    C. 41 percent
    D. 25 percent

15. A form of amnesia, lasting from seconds to days, resulting from alcohol use is a:
    A. blackout
    B. seizure
    C. convulsion
    D. delirium

16. _____ percent of all teen suicide attempts are via drug overdoses.
    A. 15 percent
    B. 73 percent
    C. 29 percent
    D. 88 percent

True or False

17. A user becomes tolerant and requires more and more of the chemicals to get the same high.

18. A slang term for amphetamines is uppers.

19. Sniffing inhalants can lead to sudden death.

20. Only the use of narcotics leads to drug addiction.

21. Withdrawal from alcohol or other depressants can result in death.

22. Cough syrups containing codeine are classified as depressants.

23. Marijuana use has been proven to result in cellular damage to the body.

24. Depressants used in combination with alcohol are not potentially fatal.

25. The repeated use of narcotics results in increased tolerance.

26. Moderate to heavy marijuana use by males results in a decreased sperm count and an abundance of abnormally formed sperm.

27. It is okay to take medication prescribed for someone else if you have similar symptoms.

28. Marijuana can be addicting.

29. People sometimes use psychoactive substances to feel part of a group.

30. When a person becomes high and drives, it is human nature that the person will become more cautious than normal.

31. If a chemically dependent person really wanted to, he/she could stop drinking or using to excess.

32. Society is very unified about the cause of psychoactive substance abuse/dependence.

33. Most chemically dependent people are men.

34. Withdrawal from narcotics produces physical discomfort but does not result in death.

35. An overdose of cannabis can produce psychosis.

36. The media does not really influence how people view using psychoactive substances.

37. Psychoactive substances get into the bloodstream almost as soon as they are ingested.

38. More teenagers die in drug- and alcohol-related motor vehicle accidents than from any disease.

39. Physical dependency means that a person would get withdrawal symptoms upon decreasing or ceasing the use of a chemical substance.

40. A person cannot become addicted to prescription drugs.

41. Once psychoactive substances enter the brain they do not circulate back through the body again.

42. Studies have shown that chronic exposure to some solvents and gasoline causes severe anemia and leukemia.

43. The effects of marijuana on female reproduction are of short duration.

44. The intravenous injection of narcotics or other substances can result in hepatitis, AIDS, or other infections from contaminated needles.

45. Two reasons why people sometimes try to persuade friends to use drugs are to see the effects on someone else or because they do not want to use alone.

46. Heavy drinking for a long period of time may cause physical problems but does not cause brain damage.

47. Dependency on crack can occur in a little as two weeks.

48. When psychoactive substances are snorted or inhaled they go directly to the brain.

49. A strong cup of coffee will sober people up after they have become high from using psychoactive substances.

50. When using stimulants, drivers tend to overreact at the wheel.

51. It is important for family members of a chemically dependent person to talk to someone about how chemical dependency has affected their lives.

52. Seventy percent of marijuana users drive while high.

53. LSD is a stimulant.

54. The effects of PCP can last for days.

ALCOHOL AND DRUG TEST ANSWER SHEET

1.	D	28.	True
2.	D	29.	True
3.	B	30.	False
4.	C	31.	False
5.	D	32.	False
6.	A	33.	False
7.	B	34.	True
8.	C	35.	True
9.	D	36.	False
10.	D	37.	True
11.	A	38.	True
12.	B	39.	True
13.	B	40.	False
14.	C	41.	False
15.	A	42.	True
16.	D	43.	False
17.	True	44.	True
18.	True	45.	True
19.	True	46.	False
20.	False	47.	True
21.	True	48.	False
22.	False	49.	False
23.	True	50.	True
24.	False	51.	True
25.	True	52.	True
26.	True	53.	False
27.	False	54.	True

Even though alcohol passes through everyone's body the same way, there are several factors which determine what effects the alcohol will have. These are:

1. how much the person drinks
2. how fast the person drinks
3. what kind of alcoholic beverage is drunk

4. how much the person weighs
5. how much the person has eaten
6. the state or condition of the body
7. how the person thinks and feels about drinking
8. where a person drinks–the setting

(1) Amount of Alcohol

The most important influence on how alcohol affects a person is how much alcohol is drunk. The more alcohol, the greater the effects. Contrary to popular opinions, whiskey is not "stronger" than beer or wine. 5 oz. wine = 12 oz. can of beer = 1 ½ shot of whiskey

(2) Speed of Drinking

The liver metabolizes alcohol (converts it to carbon dioxide and water) at the steady rate of 3/4 ounces in an hour; it circulates in the bloodstream until the liver can metabolize it. During this process of circulation, the alcohol keeps passing through the brain. Consequently, the faster alcohol is drunk, the more alcohol reaches the brain (and other body organs), producing faster, more potent effects on the drinker.

(3) Type of Beverage Consumed

Liquor is absorbed more readily than either beer or wine, and combining liquor with carbonated drinks will increase the rate even more. Water, on the other hand, dilutes alcohol and slows down the rate of absorption.

(4) Body Weight

People who weigh more are affected less by alcohol than lighter people. Heavier people have more blood and water in their bodies to diffuse the alcohol.

(5) Food

Food slows down the passage of alcohol through the stomach. Consequently, alcohol will "go to your head" if you have not eaten before drinking or eat while you drink.

(6) Body Condition

A drinker who is tired may be more influenced by the alcohol drunk than a person who is alert. An ill person may be more affected than a healthy person. Especially worthwhile to note is that alcohol plus other drugs are not simply addictive–they are multiplicative. Alcohol can have double or triple its normal sedative effects when mixed with other drugs.

(7) Thoughts and Feelings About Drinking

Experienced drinkers often develop a psychological tolerance for alcohol. On the basis of many drinking experiences, they have learned what effects alcohol has on them and can compensate for them. Along this same line, alcohol often affects a person the way he or she expects it to. When drinkers expect to get high, they are likely to do so. Also, a person's mood affects what alcohol does to them. Alcohol may make someone who is feeling unhappy more depressed, or someone cheerful even happier. Finally, where someone drinks–the setting–may affect how much they drink and how alcohol affects them. A person might drink moderately away from friends and feel the effects, whereas at a tense gathering may not feel them as readily.

(3) Short-Term Effects of Drugs: Intoxication and Hangover

Common signs of impairment include:

- sleepiness, yawning
- slurred speech
- unstable walk
- unusual clumsiness

• silly behavior
• impatience, impulsiveness
• distortions in thinking, misperceptions of reality
• boasting
• violence, more aggressiveness than usual
• more sexual aggressiveness

Because of the motor and/or cognitive functioning impairment, intoxicated persons are particularly dangerous when driving. There are four problems involved in identifying people who are too impaired to drive:

(a) Many substance users who are impaired *seem* relatively sober to others in terms of how they walk, talk, or even drive. Individuals claim to drive "better after drinking or using drugs than when sober because I am extra careful." However, while such abusers may have learned to compensate for certain chemical substance's effects, an emergency situation such as a flat tire or pedestrian suddenly appearing would leave them unable to react quickly.

(b) The *more* people use psychoactive substances, the *less* capable they are to *judge* whether they themselves are too impaired to drive. Many people who have had several drinks or have used marijuana or stimulants really believe and *feel* they are perfectly capable of driving safely. A solution to this problem is for them to accept the opinion of a trusted friend on whether they are too impaired to drive.

(c) A driver's underlying attitudes toward driving can become unexpectedly more pronounced after drinking too much or using other chemical substances. Some drivers become cautious; others become more reckless.

(d) Marijuana adds to the alcohol effect. Drinking too much alcohol can lead to nausea and vomiting. Marijuana suppresses the "vomit center" of the brain; therefore a person can drink more than the body would normally allow, leading to higher levels of intoxication. Behind the wheel of a car and independent of each other, each is dangerous. Together, they can be fatal.

Please review the possible effects of each drug listed in the Slang Terms and Symptoms of Abuse chart in Chapter 3.

A hangover is the effect, after the passage of several hours, of too much of a drug and may include: nausea and vomiting, stomach upset, headache, muscle ache, and extensive thirst. "Hangovers can interfere with the ability to think and to do school work" (Zastrow & Kirst-Ashman, 1987, p. 221).

(4) Long-Term Effects of Drugs

"Typically, adolescents begin using out of curiosity and for experimental purposes in order to escape painful feelings, conflicts and low self-esteem, and frequently because 'everyone else is doing it'" (Morrison, 1985, p. 2).

The effects from a variety of drugs used over time may include:

Physical/Biological	*Mental/Emotional*
contributes to heart disease	chronic anxiety and/or depression
contributes to cancer	paranoia
contributes to diabetes	hallucinations
cirrhosis of the liver	delusions
increased blood pressure	impaired judgment/cognitive functioning
kidney damage	memory loss
vitamin deficiencies	aggressive behavior
chromosomal damage	apathy
insomnia	
affects hormones	
loss of appetite/malnutrition	
coma	
increased tolerance	

Most important, increased use of drugs leads to abuse which can lead to addiction and/or can result in problems involving school, crime and delinquency, relationships, and money.

TERMS AND DEFINITIONS

(1) *Drug dependence:* the state produced by repeated administration of a drug that the user will engage in repeatable behavior patterns over an extended period of time with such behaviors leading to further administration of the drug.

(2) *Poly drug use:* the simultaneous or sequential use of more than one psychoactive drug for nonmedicinal purposes.

(3) *Drug abuse:* the use of a drug, including alcohol, in a manner that deviates from the approved medical or social patterns within a given culture.

(4) *Physical dependence:* an altered psychological state produced by the repeated administration of a drug, including alcohol, which necessitates the continued administration to prevent the appearance of withdrawal symptoms.

(5) *Psychological dependence:* continued, repetitive use of the drug is required to maintain emotional or psychological equilibrium.

(6) *Drug addiction:* a behavioral pattern of drug use characterized after withdrawal.

(7) *Withdrawal symptom:* any of the symptoms caused by the withdrawal of a physically addictive drug, such as tremors, sweating, chills, vomiting, seizures, and coma. Psychologically addictive drugs, when withdrawn, can produce symptoms such as deep depression, anxiety, sense of helplessness, and an inability to function.

(8) *Tolerance:* the state that develops when, after repeated administration, a given dose of a drug produces decreased effect or, conversely, when increasingly larger doses must be administered to obtain the effects observed with the original dose.

(9) *Chemical dependence:* a psychosocial, biogenetic disease; a chronic, progressive, familial, and relapsing disease that is fatal if untreated.

(5) *Recognizing Drug Problems (Morrison, 1985, pp. 3-4)*

There is a journey on which one progresses to addiction: i.e., a period of time that is spent using, abusing, and then crossing the biochemical-genetic wall (early addiction) after which one exhibits full-blown addictive disease characteristics. This journey is considerably more rapid in adolescents than in adults.

USE: There is an increased number of users, including an increased number of female users, in adolescence. Use affects all socioeconomic classes and all grade levels: The general time frame of the using stage in the journey to addiction is from one to three years for the adolescent. Characteristics seen during the using stage include the following:

- the adolescent has no experience with alcohol or drugs
- the first episode of intoxication and/or hangover may occur
- independent use is infrequent (teens rarely use alone during this early stage)

ABUSE: Use is more regular. Weekend drinking and a regular pattern of use occurs. Teens are drinking and using drugs to communicate, to relate, to belong, to be part of the group. Legal problems may begin to occur, such as DUI and possession. Hiding and lying about drugs may occur. Teens become suspicious, vague, and secretive about what they are using and how much they are using. Tolerance changes begin to occur: tolerance to the chemical rises, leading to the need for larger doses of the chemical in order to obtain the subjective effect or "high." Emotional changes are noticed; i.e., irritability, mood swings, and a lack of caring for one's self and for others.

CROSSING THE WALL: Teens drink and use to get "high." Friends gradually change to drinking and drug-oriented peers. The teen may appear in altered states of consciousness at school and work. Time spent using and abusing is increased, with evidence of preoccupation with how and where one is going to obtain the drug, and how and where one is going to use it. The purpose of use is to escape the frustration, pain, and hurt teenagers may be experiencing. Blackouts and early withdrawal symptoms begin to occur. Blackouts are drug or alcohol amnesia, not passing out. Withdrawal symptoms may occur when use is decreased or discontinued, and may masquerade as other symptoms–a GI virus or flu, mood wings, irritability, or anxiety. More difficulties begin to occur at home and family conflict increases. Suspensions at school may occur and grades become affected. Guilt and anxiety may be experienced because of the loss of control of drug use. Adolescents become fearful and at certain levels recognize that they are hurting and cannot stop using chemicals despite negative consequences that are beginning to occur. In response to all of the above, repeated promises to stop using are made.

DISEASE: In summary, the disease of chemical dependence has the following characteristics:

(1) It is a primary, unique, and individualized disease; therefore, it is not a result of a bad habit, mental illness, lack of willpower, or stupidity. It is a primary disease entity in itself.

(2) It makes no difference how long one uses, what chemical is used, or what dose is used. One may become just as addicted with low doses as with high doses.

(3) The basic defect is biochemical and genetic. There are abnormal chemical and metabolic changes that occur in the addict to cause him/her to have the irrational, illogical compulsion to use chemicals.

(4) The chief symptom of the disease is the compulsion (or the repeated, irresistible urge) to use the chemical: i.e., continued chemical use despite consequences experienced.

(5) It is a family disease that affects every member of the family of the dependent individual.

(6) It is a progressive, chronic, and multidisciplinary disease with potential for relapse.

(6) Motivations for Drug Use and Drug Behavior

Adolescence is a time of identity search. Teenagers attempt to define their self-concept through experimenting with their appearance (clothes, hairstyles, make-up), with roles (student, child, employee, girl/boyfriend), and with hobbies and interests (music, cheerleading, sports, school newspaper, etc.) (Zastrow & Kirst-Ashman, 1987, p. 200). Experimentation may also be manifested in less healthy ways such as sexual activity, criminal behavior, or drug use.

Adolescents also attempt to achieve a sense of identity by becoming more autonomous from their parents. This autonomy not only gives them the opportunity to separate their own identity from that of their parents, but it gives them the chance to interact with those who are engaging in a similar metamorphosis. However, the adolescent's quest for autonomy may not be a comfortable situation for parents who do not understand the adolescent's need to be independent. This results in conflict. As Morrison (1985, p. 1) says, "Impaired parental-adolescent interaction, ranging from attitudes of parental rejection to overprotection may lead to difficulties in communication and relationships." Thus, the adolescent may act out at her/his parents, whom she/he perceives as not understanding– and who actually may not be understanding–by taking drugs.

Morrison (1985, p. 1) says about adolescence that "during this time when teens are no longer children but not yet adults, adult demands begin to be placed on individuals who have the maturity level of a child." Adolescence is a time of mixed messages and the teen may ask, "Am I an adult or not?" If he/she is being treated like an adult, then why cannot he/she act like an adult by, say, drinking, as do his/her adult parents? Thus, parental modeling, even that which is unintentional, is another motivation for drug use.

Morrison (1985, p. 1) states another reason for possible drug use. "Various situations, crises, or traumatic events, such as parental divorce, separation, death, loss, move, or illness, may also present problems for the adolescent."

In addition, because the teen spends more time with his/her peers and, through the struggle for identity, wants to be like everyone else, peer pressure may be a motivation for drug use. Simultaneously there is pressure from high-sales pitches on television, radio, in popular magazines, and in popular music.

These motivations for drug use will be dealt with more specifically in Week II.

WEEK II

(1) Continuation of Topics

Please review last week's session and ask questions on anything about which you are unclear.

(2) Brief Presentation About Social Learning of Substance Abuse

Briefly stated, the social learning theory posits that we learn behaviors by observing other people. As Vender Zanden (1978) explains:

> . . . if we learned solely by direct experience–by the rewarding and punishing consequences of our behavior–most of us would not survive to adulthood. If, for example, we depended upon direct conditioning to learn how to cross the street, most of us would already be traffic fatalities . . . we avoid tedious, costly, trial-and-error experimentation by imitating the behavior of socially competent models. (p. 80)

Unfortunately, not all models from whom we learn are "socially competent," nor are the behaviors we learn always positive or adaptive. The use of drugs and/or alcohol is one such learned behavior.

Albert Bandura (1977), a foremost social learning theorist, demonstrated in several research experiments that children learn aggressive behavior through observation. Adolescents, likewise, learn behaviors by imitating what they see in the media, what they see in the home, and what they see their friends doing.

America is a drug culture. In movies, on television, and in the lyrics of songs, the message is that drug use is popular, that it is "cool."

> Americans are obsessed with taking pills . . . drug companies spend millions in advertising to convince customers that they are too tense, too irritable, take too long to fall asleep, that they should lose weight, and so on. These companies then assert their medications will relieve these problems. (Zastrow & Kirst-Ashman, 1987, p. 222)

Advertisements for alcohol, especially, abound using catchy slogans ("Gimme a light–Bud Light!," "It's Miller time!"), cutesy mascots (the Budweiser Clydesdale horses, "Spuds MacKenzie"), and popular celebrities (Mark Harmon, Bruce Willis) to enhance its appeal.

Adolescence, with its tribulations and confusion, presents for most teens a period of rather intense vulnerability, when persons are easily influenced and persuaded. Thus, the media can be a particularly powerful means of conveying the message that "drugs are okay."

Parental modeling, even that which is unintentional, may be another means by which adolescents learn to drink or use drugs. Often, teens witness their parents drinking, smoking cigarettes, or taking prescription or over-the-counter medications and assume that, because someone they view as an otherwise positive role model is engaging in this behavior, then it must be a good thing to do. The implicit message the teen receives is, "Here is a positive role model. She/he is someone I respect and admire. She or he has taught me many essential, positive behaviors by being a model. Here she/he is drinking/smoking cigarettes, etc. If she/he does it, then it is okay for me to do it, too."

Furthermore, most parents who engage in such behaviors forbid their teens to do the same by threat of punishment. Because teens see their parents doing one thing, but hear something else, they become confused. As Vander Zanden (1978) says, "The command 'Do as I say, not as I do,' boomerangs. People are more influenced by the model's behavior–the 'as I do' part of the command–than by the reinforcement or the punishment associated with the 'as I say' part" (p. 82). Thus, the teen is likely to experiment with alcohol or drugs anyway because he/she *sees* Mom and/or Dad doing it.

Peer pressure is an especially potent means of influencing the use of drugs and alcohol. Because adolescence is a time of trying to "fit in" and feel good about oneself, adolescents want to do what their friends are doing. Peers may, in fact, be more influential than parents because adolescence is a time when persons begin emotionally, at least, to "leave the nest" and bond with those outside of the family. Moreover, teens receive ". . . subsequent reinforcement [to drink] by significant peers . . ." (Wodarski, 1987b, p. 127). For example, "locker room talk" revolving around bragging about how much one drank over the weekend is often rewarded through praise and acceptance, therefore increasing the likelihood that such behavior will occur again.

Still another reason for drug and/or alcohol use is what some believe to be positive rewarding effects of these substances. As Wodarski (1987a, p. 127) says, "Social learning theorists emphasize that the abuse of alcohol is learned from the consequences that follow drinking. These most often include (1) stress reduction, (2) removal from an unpleasant situation, (3) an excuse for otherwise unacceptable behavior, and (4) the need to escape from thought of academic failure."

To summarize, adolescents learn to use drugs/alcohol because of the powerful influence of the media, because of parental modeling (even that which is unintentional or unconscious), because of peer pressure to do so and acceptance by these peers when the behavior is engaged in, and because of the learned consequences–often perceived as positive–of drinking or using drugs such as escape from problems and reduction of tension.

Exercise One (adapted from Zastrow & Kirst-Ashman, 1987, pp. 220-221)

Consider the following scenarios and discuss.

Scene: Jane, a 16-year-old high school sophomore, likes to go out with friends and drink beer. She thinks it is okay; after all, Mom and Dad have been to quite a few parties or entertained in their own home and alcohol was served.

Scene: Tom, age 17, thought getting drunk was great; it relieved his anxiety about school and, best of all, helped him forget the problems between his parents. Besides, drinking is what his father did every time he had a fight with his wife, or when things were bad at work.

Scene: 14-year-old Pam almost could not wait for Saturday and the big party. Everyone who was anyone was going to be there. Saturday night arrived and she and her best friend Susie went together. Once there, they noticed some older kids who were passing around marijuana. These kids encouraged Pam and Susie to join them, which Susie did. Pam did not know what to do. She was afraid to smoke the marijuana because she knew it might be harmful, yet she did not want to look like a nerd.

Exercise Two

Discuss ways in which teens receive "It's okay to use drugs/ drink" messages through the media, in music, and through popular role models (i.e., celebrities). Also, examine ways in which these influences are and can be altered to present healthy, positive attitudes and messages and be used to warn about the dangers of drug/alcohol use.

(3) Presentation of Parents' Role in Helping Change Behavior and Support for Behavior Change

There are several areas to consider when examining ways you as a parent can help change behavior and give support for behavioral change, especially that behavior associated with drug/alcohol use.

You have taken a first step by educating yourself to alcohol/drug types, their effects, and the use/abuse/addiction pattern, among other things. Educating your teen(s) as to drug and alcohol effects and dangers is also important.

Secondly, it is important for you to realize, as Wodarski (1987a) has learned in studying adolescents that,

> . . . students can change or determine behavior by altering the environment, be it internal or external. The two major categories of environmental events that must be understood and manipulated to produce the desired outcome are: events that precede and set the stage for particular behavior, and events that follow the behavior and make them more or less likely to reoccur (Williams & Long, 1979). Thus, one learning experience is to help students identify environmental events controlling behavior and then alter the ones necessary to produce the desired behaviors. Examples of external environmental stimuli that cue drinking behavior are parties or peer statements. Examples of internal environmental events are emotional upset and loneliness. (p. 128)

Thus, as a parent, you can help your adolescent change her/his behavior by teaching her/him how to alter the environment through self-management skills such as learned assertiveness, meaningful interaction with others, and effective coping strategies for everyday problems (Wodarski, 1987a).

As a parent, you will learn in the sessions that follow about effective parent-adolescent communication skills, the problem-solving method, and assertiveness training.

As Zastrow and Kirst-Ashman (1987) have noted, "Keeping the lines of communication open is admittedly easier said than done. It requires work!" (p. 243). Week III will give you a chance to learn effective communication techniques and provide you with an opportunity to practice them in role-play exercises. You will also learn, in Week IV, the basics of the problem-solving method, which is ". . . a cooperative way of approaching conflict in which the parties attempt to find a solution that satisfies everyone" (Auvine et al., 1978, p. 48). Week V will teach you assertiveness training and provide you with an opportunity to practice all that you have learned up until then.

WEEK III

(1) What Is Communication?

The most important thing for parents to keep in mind, at any time or any age of the child, is not to say anything that will break down or cut off the lines of communication between parent and child. All teenagers need help, even if they do not recognize this need or seem grateful for it. They must feel free to seek that help from their parents or loved ones. If teenagers cannot talk to their parents or to other acceptable adults, they have only their peers and friends to turn to. How much advice and information on serious matters can one 13-year-old or 15-year-old give to another? (Kaluger & Kaluger, 1984, p. 370; quoted in Zastrow & Kirst-Ashman, 1987, p. 243).

The following is *not* a test. However, in order to help you better understand the communication patterns between you and your adolescent(s), it will be helpful for you to read over the questionnaire. Please spend a few minutes jotting down answers to each question. When everyone has completed the questionnaire, we will spend some time discussing the responses. You are not required to volunteer your answers. However, please remember that it is the sharing of ideas that will enable everyone to learn about more effective communication.

QUESTIONNAIRE

Place a check mark (✔) under "Yes" if it tends to be true, and under "No" if it tends not to be true.

YES   *NO*

_____   _____   1. We have open and effective communication in our home.

_____   _____   2. My teen(s) seem(s) to feel comfortable discussing things with me.

_____   _____   3. We *never* disagree or have conflicts in our family.

_____   _____   4. In our home, the adolescent(s) make(s) the decisions about the rules, responsibilities, punishments, etc.

_____   _____   5. I tend to be overly critical when my adolescent(s) make(s) mistakes.

_____   _____   6. In our home, virtually any topic is allowable for conversation.

_____   _____   7. I often tell my teen(s) I'm listening to him/her/them when actually I'm preoccupied by the TV, newspaper, a task I'm working on, or a problem of my own.

_____   _____   8. When I correct my adolescent(s) for a wrong-doing, I make sure I criticize the *action*, not him/her/them.

_____   _____   9. I believe an adolescent should be seen and not heard.

_____   _____   10. I praise my teen(s) not only for a "job well done," but also for just making the effort.

_____   _____   11. My teen(s) and I have regular times when we sit down and discuss things.

SHORT ANSWER

12. What do you feel you do best when talking with your teen(s)? What are the most effective things you do when having a discussion?

13. What do you feel are the least effective "techniques" you use when talking with your teen(s)? What are areas in which you need improvement?

Take a few minutes to discuss your answers to the preceding questionnaire.

Consider the following scenario (Wodarski and Wodarski, 1993).

> It is a nasty, rainy day outside. Your 13-year-old teenager, ready for school, heads for the door without even a raincoat. You ask her about wearing a raincoat, and are concerned that she might catch a cold without one.

Divide up into pairs, one role-playing the adolescent and one the parent. Role-play a conversation between the two. Take about ten minutes. Switch roles and repeat the same scenario for an additional ten minutes. When all pairs have completed the role-play, get back in the large group and discuss how each person, as the parent, handled the situation.

(2) Parent-Adolescent Communication

A. *Keeping the Lines of Communication Open*

You do this by remembering the following (quoted from *Helping Your Child to Say "NO" to Alcohol,* National Institute on Alcohol Abuse and Alcoholism, 1986, p. 11):

–Don't make any subjects off limits. Your kids feel they can talk to you about anything, from alcohol to sex to clothing to hockey. If you always change the subject, come down hard on the subject (or your child) right away, or lose your temper, he/she won't approach you.

–Listen "between the lines." A child who comes home and says,

"Tom's dad lets him have a beer on Friday nights," wants to know how you feel about the idea. You are being tested. You may feel like saying, "That's the most ridiculous thing I've ever heard of, and if I catch you doing that I'll break your legs." Do yourself a favor, instead . . .

–Get the conversation moving. In a calm voice say, "What would you do if Tom's dad offered you a beer?" Situations like this offer your child a chance to express his/her worries, and give you a chance to provide helpful suggestions for handling problems. Keeping it hypothetical ("What *would* you do *if* . . .") makes it easier for your teen to talk to you.

B. *Nonverbal Communication*

Body language or nonverbal behavior includes any bodily and/or facial movements involved in communication. Proven in research studies to ". . . strongly influence interactions between people . . .," nonverbal behaviors may be more potent in revealing underlying feelings that are actual words (Hepsworth & Larsen, 1986, pp. 83-84).

Kids pick up on the silent vibes parents send. For instance, if your child wants to talk to you and you are reading or watching TV, put down the paper or shut off the tube. Focus on your child. Direct eye contact means, "I'm listening. You have my full attention" (*Helping Your Child to Say "NO,"* National Institute on Alcohol Abuse and Alcoholism, 1986, p. 11).

Thus, parents need to monitor their own nonverbal behaviors, including eye contact, tone of voice, body posture, and facial expressions.

The most effective body language includes:

• Maintaining direct eye contact (except where in cultures this is considered rude or inappropriate).

• A body posture that is open, meaning that the arms and legs are relaxed (as opposed to arms and legs being tightly crossed as in a defensive manner).

• Using facial expressions that are expressive (such as head nods) and that are consistent with what your teen is saying (i.e., smiling when something positive is said, or showing concern when pain is expressed).

• Using a tone of voice that is congruent with what is being said.

Parents can, by being aware of their own body language, learn to be more cognizant of their adolescent's nonverbal behavior.

It is important for parents to remember when assessing their own, as well as their adolescent's, body language that, when there is inconsistency between body language and what is said (for example, the teen says nothing is wrong, yet will not look you in the eye and has tightly crossed arms), the body language more accurately conveys the real meaning of the message.

C. *Ineffective Verbal Communication* (For an elaboration of the techniques described below see *PET Instructor's Manual*, Gordon, 1975, pp. B3-B6.)

Gordon (1975) has identified 12 roadblocks to effective communication and four skills for effective communication with your adolescent. The 12 roadblocks are ordering, warning or threatening, moralizing, advising or suggesting, teaching or lecturing, judging or critizing, praising, name-calling or labeling, interpreting or analyzing, reassuring or sympathizing, probing or questioning, and withdrawing or distracting. For example, ordering is considered a roadblock because it tells or commands the child to do something, such as "Don't talk to your mother like that!" or "I don't care what other children do, you have to do the yard work!"

The four skills for effective communicating are silence, noncommittal acknowledgement, door openers, and feedback or reflecting. A door opener, for example, might be "Tell me about it," or "I'd be interested in what you have to say," where one conveys an invitation to say more about a subject or situation.

D. *Expressing Affection/Giving Praise and Compliments*

Affection can be infectious. A parent can't give too many hugs, kisses, or pats on the back. It's important to show your kids that you love them. (*Helping Your Child to Say "NO,"* 1986, p. 13)

It is also important to compliment your teen for things done right. Additionally, the effort your teen puts forth, whether or not it results in success, should likewise be praised. Parents might want to remember the old adage–"it's not whether you win or lose, but how you play the game."

Giving praise and compliments as described herein should not be confused with the roadblock to effective communication described previously. In that instance, praise is inappropriate because it attempts to smooth over situations and thus blocks your teen's expression of feelings. Here, however, we are describing praise and compliments given unconditionally as a sign that you love and respect your teen.

E. *Negotiating and Reaching Agreements Before Terminating Discussion*

> Parent Effectiveness Training (P.E.T.) skills . . . employ a 'no-lose' method of resolving conflicts. It is a no-power method; conflicts are resolved with no one winning and no one losing. Both win because the solution must be acceptable to both. Parents and adolescents encounter a conflict-of-needs situation. The parent asks the adolescent to participate with him/her in a joint search for some solution acceptable to both. One or both may offer possible solutions. They critically evaluate them and eventually make a decision on a final solution acceptable to both. No selling of the other is required after the solution has been selected because both have already accepted it. No power is required to force compliance because neither is resisting the decision. (Wodarski and Wodarski, 1993)

In this way, parents and teens can negotiate and reach agreements in a healthy, productive manner and without risking ending a conversation on an abrupt note with conflicts left unresolved.

Remember the scenario described earlier in which you took turns role-playing the parent? Examine the conversation between parent and adolescent (p. 176) as an *example* of effective communication, and discuss the components and specific elements found in this scenario.

the

"I" message

book

THE "I" MESSAGE BOOK

The 3 parts of "I" messages:

1. I feel _____
(an emotion)

2. when you _____
(action of others)

3. because _____
(how action affects you)

1

Words for expressing ANGER

annoyed	teed off
put out	bugged
upset with	pissed off
irritated	resentful
burned	furious

Words for expressing CONFUSION

uneasy	uncomfortable
bothered	unsure
uncertain	disturbed
frustrated	lost
troubled	mixed-up
puzzled	ambivalent

Words for expressing HURT

taken for granted	let down
	put down
unappreciated	used
neglected	betrayed
mistreated	crushed
criticized	
wounded	

Words for expressing ANXIETY

insecure	self-conscious
worried	uncomfortable
shy	awkward
shaky	nervous
tense	uptight
defensive	scared
afraid	desperate

2

3

DIRECTIONS:

1. Cut along solid lines so that you have eight pages.
2. Put pages in order and staple along left edge.
3. Write any additional feeling words you can think of on the backs of the printed pages.

Words for expressing INADEQUACY

uncertain	unimportant
small	incapable
clumsy	stupid
inferior	like a failure
helpless	worthless

Words for expressing DEPRESSION

sad	down
low	unhappy
lousy	gloomy
hopeless	awful
rotten	miserable

4

Words for expressing GUILT

blew it	goofed
at fault	wrong
silly	ridiculous
foolish	ashamed
horrible	humiliated
unforgivable	sick at heart

Words for expressing LONELINESS

excluded	left out
shut out	alone
rejected	alienated
cut off	isolated

5

Words for expressing STRENGTH

can cope	up to it
important	in control
successful	capable
able	effective
committed	inspired
determined	confident

Words for expressing HAPPINESS

calm	fulfilled
satisfied	good
wonderful	super
enthusiastic	excited
terrific	fantastic

6

Words for expressing LOVE

accept	like
friendly	value
trust	concern for
admire	respect
fond of	affection for
devoted to	cherish

7

PARENT EFFECTIVENESS TRAINING SCENARIO

Jane: Bye, I'm off to school.

Father: Honey, it's raining outside and you don't have your raincoat on.

Jane: I don't need it.

Father: I think it's raining quite hard and I'm concerned that you'll ruin your clothes or get a cold, and that will affect us.

Jane: Well, I sure don't want to wear my raincoat.

Father: You sure sound like you definitely don't want to wear that raincoat.

Jane: That's right, I hate it.

Father: You really hate your raincoat.

Jane: Yeah, it's plaid.

Father: Something about plaid raincoats you hate, huh?

Jane: Yes, nobody at school wears plaid raincoats.

Father: You don't want to be the only one wearing something different.

Jane: I sure don't. Everybody wears plain-colored raincoats–either white or blue or green.

Father: I see. Well, we really have a conflict here. You don't want to wear your raincoat 'cause it's plaid, but I sure don't want to pay a cleaning bill, and I will not feel comfortable with you getting a cold. Can you think of a solution that we both could accept? How could we solve this so we're both happy?

Jane: (pause) Maybe I could borrow Mom's car coat today.

Father: What does that look like? Is it plain-colored?

Jane: Yeah, it's white.

Father: Think she'll let you wear it today?

Jane: I'll ask her. (Comes back in a few minutes with car coat on; sleeves are too long, but she rolls them back.) It's OK by Mom.

Father: You're happy with that thing?

Jane: Sure, it's fine.

Father: Well, I'm convinced it will keep you dry. So if you're happy with that solution, I am too.

Jane: Well, so long.

Father: So long. Have a good day at school.

What happened here? Obviously, Jane and her father resolved their conflict to the mutual satisfaction of both. It was resolved rather quickly, too. The father did not have to waste time being an imploring salesman, trying to sell his solution. No power was involved–either on the part of the father or of Jane. Finally, both walked away from the problem solving feeling warm toward each other. The father could say, "Have a good day at school" and really mean it, and Jane could go to school free of the fear of embarrassment over a plaid raincoat.

WEEK IV

(1) Continuation of Topics

Please review last week's session and ask questions on anything about which you are unclear.

(2) The Problem-Solving Method

Zastrow and Kirst-Ashman (1987) explain typical parent-adolescent exchanges in the following:

> In every parent-teenager relationship there are inevitable situations where the youth continues to behave in a way that interferes with the needs of the parent. Conflict is a part of life and not

necessarily bad. Conflict is bound to occur because people are different and have different needs and wants, which at times do not match. What is important is not how frequently conflicts arise, but how the conflicts get resolved. Generally, in a conflict between parent and youth, a power struggle is created.

In many families the power struggle is resolved by one of two win-lose approaches. Most parents try to resolve the conflict by having the parent winning and the youth losing. . . . In other families, . . . the win-lose conflict is resolved by the parents giving in to their teenagers out of fear of frustrating them or fear of conflict. (pp. 244-245)

Dr. Thomas Gordon (1975) has devised the no-lose problem-solving method which has two premises: ". . . (a) that all people have the right to get their needs met and (b) that what is in conflict between the two parties involved is not their *needs* but their *solutions* to those needs" (Gordon, as quoted in Zastrow & Kirst-Ashman, 1987, p. 245).

On the next page are listed the six steps to the problem-solving method. Take a few minutes to look over these, then discuss them. Notice that the page can be cut out and folded into a bookmark for handy reference.

(3) Application of the Problem-Solving Method

Collision of values are common between parents and their children, particularly as the children become adolescents and young adults. Likely areas of conflict include values about sexual behavior, clothing, religion, choice of friends, education, plans for the future, use of drugs, hairstyles, and eating habits. In these areas emotions run strong and parents generally seek to influence their offspring to follow the values the parents hold as important. Teenagers, on the other hand, often think their parents' values are old fashioned and stupid, and declare that they want to make their own decisions about these matters. (Zastrow & Kirst-Ashman, 1987, p. 245)

Consider the common scenario on page 114, and discuss the components of the problem-solving method found in this situation.

THE PROBLEM-SOLVING
METHOD

STEP 1
State the problem

STEP 2
Identify needs

STEP 3
Brainstorm

STEP 4
List pros and cons

STEP 5
Try a solution

STEP 6
Evaluate the outcome

THE PROBLEM-SOLVING
METHOD

STEP 1
What is the problem?
Write it down.

STEP 2
What are your needs?
What needs of others
are involved?

STEP 3
Write down as many
alternatives as you
can think of.
Be creative!

STEP 4
Consider the likely
outcome of each
alternative.

STEP 5
Pick the alternative
that seems the most
promising, then
carry it out.

STEP 6
Did it work?
If not, try another.

fold here

When you have discussed this scenario, return to this page for a continuation of our current discussion.

With the example on page 114 in mind, break up into groups of three for role-playing exercises. Each of you will take turns playing the teenager, parent, and observer. (The observer's function is to give feedback). After about ten minutes in a role, switch roles. The following are sample problem situations of interpersonal relationships for the scenarios:

(a) Discussing chemical/substance use (including alcohol) with your teen; include such topics as driving, harmful effects of use, etc.

(b) Asking the adolescent to carry out simple chores (i.e., cutting the grass, doing the dishes, taking out the trash).

(c) Discussing school experiences (grades, teachers, peers, extracurricular activities, etc.).

(d) Discussing sexuality with your adolescent.

Each group should attempt to complete role-playing exercises in two out of these four sample situations (all members thus will play the teen twice in two different scenes, the parent twice, etc.). Because the focus of this training seminar is substance use, all group members are asked to complete a scenario involving problem situation (a).

After role-playing exercise, please take some time discussing how it felt/how you reacted in each role. Also, discuss the techniques you used, their effectiveness, what you could have done differently to make your efforts more effective, and so forth.

PROBLEM-SOLVING METHOD SCENARIO

Mother: Cindy, I'm sick and tired of nagging you about your room, and I'm sure you're tired of my getting on your back about it. Every once in a while you clean it up, but mostly it's a mess and I'm mad. Let's try a new method I've learned in class. Let's see if we can find a solution we both will accept—one that will make us both happy. I don't want to make you clean your room and have you be unhappy with that, but I don't want to be embarrassed and uncomfortable and be mad at you either. How could we solve this problem once and for all? Will you try?

Cindy: Well, I'll try but I know I'll just end up having to keep it clean.

Mother: No. I am suggesting we find a solution that would definitely be acceptable to both, not just to me.

Cindy: Well, I've got an idea. You hate to cook but like cleaning and I hate cleaning and love to cook. And besides I want to learn more about cooking. What if I cook two dinners a week for you and Dad and me if you clean up my room once or twice a week?

Mother: Do you think that would work out, really?

Cindy: Yes, I'd really love it.

Mother: OK, then let's give it a try. Are you also offering to do the dishes?

Cindy: Sure.

Mother: OK. Maybe now your room will get cleaned according to my own standards. After all, I'll be doing it myself.

WEEK V

(1) Assertiveness Training

There are three basic styles of interpersonal behavior (Wodarski and Wodarski, 1993):

     a. Aggressive style–fighting, accusing, threatening, and generally stepping on people without regard for their feelings.
     b. Passive style–when a person lets others push one around, when one does not stand up for oneself, and when one does what one is told regardless of how one feels about it.
     c. Assertive style–a person stands up for oneself, expresses one's true feelings, and does not let others take advantage of him/her. At the same time, one is considerate of others' feelings.

Assertiveness training can be important for parents and teens alike, since interacting ". . . with others can be a source of stress in one's life. Assertiveness training can reduce that stress by teaching one to stand up for his/her legitimate rights without bullying others or letting them bully him/her" (Wodarski and Wodarski, 1993).

Consider the following scenarios (Wodarski and Wodarski, 1993). Label each one as an example of aggressive, passive, or assertive style. The answers are at the end of the last scenario.

Scene 1

    A. Is that a new dent I see in the car?

    B. Look, I just got home, it was a wretched day and I don't want to talk about it now.

    A. This is important to me, and we're going to talk about it now!

    B. Have a heart.

    A. Let's decide now who is going to pay to have it fixed, when, and where.

    B. I'll take care of it. Now leave me alone, for heaven's sake!

Scene 2

    A. You left me so by myself at the party . . . I really felt abandoned.

    B. You were being a party pooper.

    A. I didn't know anybody–the least you could have done is introduce me to some of your friends.

    B. Listen, you're grown up. You can take care of yourself. I'm tired of your nagging to be taken care of all the time.

    A. And I'm tired of your inconsiderateness.

    B. Okay, I'll stick to you like glue next time.

Scene 3

A. Would you mind helping me for a minute with this file?

B. I'm busy with this report. Catch me later.

A. Well, I really hate to bother you, but it's important.

B. Look, I have a four o'clock deadline.

A. Okay, I understand. I know it's hard to be interrupted.

Scene 4

A. I got a letter from Mom this morning. She wants to come and spend two weeks with us. I'd really like to see her.

B. Oh no, not your mother! And right on the heels of your sister. When do we get a little time to ourselves?

A. Well, I do want her to come, but I know you need to spend some time without in-laws under foot. I'd like to invite her to come in a month, and instead of two weeks, I think one week would be enough. What do you say to that?

B. That's a big relief to me.

Scene 5

A. Boy, you're looking great today!

B. Who do you think you're kidding? My hair is a fright and my clothes aren't fit for the Goodwill box.

A. Have it your way.

B. And I feel just as bad as I look today.

A. Right. I've got to run now.

Scene 6

> (While at a party, A is telling her friends how much she appreciates her boyfriend taking her out to good restaurants and to the theater. Her friends criticize her for being unliberated.)

A. Not so; I don't make nearly as much as a secretary as he does as a lawyer. I couldn't afford to take us both out or pay my own way at all the nice places we go. Certain traditions make sense, given the economic realities.

Answer Key

Scene 1: A is aggressive. A's initial hostile statement indicates resentment and withdrawal.

Scene 2: A is aggressive. The tone is accusing and blaming. B is immediately placed on the defensive and no one wins.

Scene 3: A is passive. A's timid opening line is followed by complete collapse. The file problem must be dealt with alone.

Scene 4: A is assertive. The request is specific, non-hostile, open to negotiation and successful.

Scene 5: A is passive. A allows the compliment to be rebuffed and surrenders to B's rush of negativity.

Scene 6: A is assertive. She stands up to the prevailing opinion of the group and achieves a clear, non-threatening statement of her position.

Now take a few minutes looking over and discussing the LADDER and Mistaken Traditional Assumptions and Legitimate Rights on the next four pages.

LADDER

The first letters of each element combine to spell "LADDER." You may find this a useful mnemonic device to recall the steps toward assertive behavior. The LADDER script can be used to rewrite your problem scenes so that you can assert what you want. Initially, LADDER scripts should be written out and practiced well in advance of the problem situation for which they are created. Writing the script forces you to clarify your needs, and increases your confidence in success.

As an example of a ladder script, let's say that Jean wants to assert her right to half an hour each day of uninterrupted peace and quiet while she does her relaxation exercises. Frank often interrupts with questions and attention-getting maneuvers. Jean's script goes like this:

Look at: It's my responsibility to make sure Frank respects my needs, and I am certainly entitled to some time to myself.

Arrange: I'll ask him if he's willing to discuss this problem when he gets home tonight. If he isn't, we'll set a time and place to talk about it in the next day or so.

Define: At least once, and sometimes more often, I'm interrupted during my relaxation exercises–even though I've shut the door and asked for the time to myself. My concentration is broken and it becomes harder to achieve the relaxation.

Describe: I feel angry when my time alone is broken into, and frustrated that the exercises are then made more difficult.

Express: I would like not to be interrupted, except in dire emergency, when my door is closed. As long as it is closed, assume that I am still doing the exercises and want to be alone.

Reinforce: If I'm not interrupted, I'll come in afterward and chat with you. If I am interrupted, it will increase the time I take doing the exercises.

As another example, Harold has felt very reluctant to approach his boss to find out why he was turned down for a promotion. He's received no feedback about the reasons for the decision, and Harold is now feeling somewhat negative toward the company, and his boss in particular. Harold's script is as follows:

*L*ook at: Resentment won't solve this. I need to assert my right to reasonable feedback from my employer.

*A*rrange: I'll send him a memo tomorrow morning asking for time to discuss this problem.

*D*efine: I haven't gotten any feedback about the promotion. The position I applied for has been filled by someone else, and that's all I know.

*D*escribe: I felt uncomfortable not knowing why I didn't get it and how the decision was made.

*E*xpress: So I'd like to get some feedback from you about how my performance was seen, and what went into the decision.

*R*einforce: I think your feedback will help me do a better job.

These scripts are specific and detailed. The statement of the problem is clear and to the point, without blaming, accusing, or being passive. The feelings are expressed with "I" messages and are linked to specific events or behaviors, not to evaluations of Jean's husband or Harold's boss. "I" messages provide a tremendous amount of safety for the assertive individual because they usually keep the other person from getting defensive and angry. You are not accusing anyone of being a bad person, you are merely stating what you want or feel entitled to.

Successful LADDER scripts to the following:

1. When appropriate, establish a mutually agreeable time and place to assert your needs.
2. Describe behavior objectively, without judging or devaluing.
3. Describe clearly, using specific references to time, place, and frequency.

4. Express feelings calmly and directly.
5. Confine your feeling response to the specific problem behavior, not the whole person.
6. Avoid delivering put-downs disguised as "honest feelings."
7. Ask for changes that are reasonably possible, and small enough not to incur a lot of resistance.
8. Ask for no more than one or two very specific changes at a time.
9. Make the reinforcements explicit, offering something that is really desirable to the other person.
10. Avoid punishments that are too big to be more than idle threats.
11. Keep your mind on your rights and goals when being assertive.

Mistaken Traditional Assumptions and Legitimate Rights

Mistaken Traditional Assumptions	Your Legitimate Rights
1. It is selfish to put your needs before others' needs.	You have a right to put yourself first sometimes.
2. It is shameful to make mistakes. You should have an appropriate response for every occasion.	You have a right to make mistakes.
3. If you cannot convince others that your feelings are reasonable, then they must be wrong, or maybe you are going crazy.	You have a right to be the final judge of your feelings and accept them as legitimate.
4. You should respect the views of others, especially if they are in a position of authority. Keep your differences of opinion to yourself. Listen and learn.	You have a right to have your own opinions and convictions.
5. You should always try to be logical and consistent.	You have a right to change your mind or decide on a different course of action.
6. You should be flexible and adjust. Others have good reasons for their actions and it's not polite to question them.	You have a right to protest unfair treatment or criticism.

7. You should never interrupt people. Asking questions reveals your stupidity to others.

You have a right to interrupt in order to ask for clarification.

8. Things could get even worse, do not rock the boat.

You have a right to negotiate for change.

9. You should not take up others' valuable time with your problems.

You have a right to ask for help or emotional support.

10. People do not want to hear that you feel bad, so keep it to yourself.

You have a right to feel and express pain.

11. When someone takes the time to give you advice, you should take it very seriously. She/he is often right.

You have a right to ignore the advice of others.

12. Knowing that you did something well is its own reward. People do not like show-offs. Successful people are secretly disliked and envied. Be modest when complimented.

You have a right to receive formal recognition for your work and achievements.

13. You should always try to accommodate others. If you do not, they will not be there when you need them.

You have a right to say "no."

14. Do not be anti-social. People are going to think you do not like them if you say you would rather be alone instead of with them.

You have a right to be alone, even if others would prefer your company.

15. You should always have a good reason for what you feel and do.

You have a right not to have to justify yourself to others.

16. When someone is in trouble, you should help them.

You have a right not to take responsibility for someone else's problem.

17. You should be sensitive to the needs and wishes of others, even when they are unable to tell you what they want.

You have a right not to have to anticipate others' needs and wishes.

18. It is always a good policy to stay on people's good side.	You have a right not to always worry about the goodwill of others.
19. It is not nice to put people off. If questioned, give an answer.	You have a right to choose not to respond to a situation.

(2) Overview and Practice of Skills

Think back on areas of previous conflict you have had with your adolescent concerning substance use/abuse, or imagine one that might come up. With three persons to a group, role-play as you have done previously in these sessions. Try to role-play with different persons than you have previously. Incorporate the things we have discussed in these sessions, including your knowledge of substances/effects/differences between uses and abuses; social learning theory and abuse; effective communication techniques; the problem-solving method; and assertiveness training. This is a lot to remember; so, before proceeding take ten to fifteen minutes to look back over prior material.

At the end of the role-play exercise, discuss how you handled the problem this time as compared to how you would have handled it previously. Also, use this time to ask any questions about anything discussed during these sessions.

(3) Wrap-Up and Feedback

The instructor will be present to receive feedback from you on your perception of the effectiveness of these exercises and to close the sessions.

SUMMARY

This chapter has elucidated a paradigm that can be utilized to involve parents in order to support the acquisition of knowledge and relevant social behaviors in their adolescents. It is emphasized that the procedures need to be concrete and teach specific ways that parents can provide support. Moreover, the delivery of the content should be accomplished in an attractive facilitative manner and usually completed in five two-hour sessions. A program that does not include the parents to support adolescents in developing the knowledge about substances and requisite preventive behaviors has a lesser probability of being successful.

The following are sources of additional information on alcohol and drug use/abuse:

National Council on Alcoholism
12 West 21st Street
7th Floor
New York, NY 10010
(212) 206-6770

National Federation of Parents for Drug-Free Youth
8730 Georgia Avenue
Suite 200
Silver Spring, MD 20910
1-800-554-KIDS

National Parents Resource Institute on Drug Education (PRIDE)
Robert W. Woodruff Volunteer Service Center
Suite 1002
100 Edgewood Avenue
Atlanta, GA 30303
(404) 658-2548

The National Clearinghouse for Alcohol Information
P.O. Box 2345
Rockville, MD 20852
(301) 468-2600

REFERENCES

Auvine, B., Densmore, B., Extrom, M., Poole, S., Shanklin, M. (1978). *A Manual for Group Facilitators.* Madison, WI: The Center for Conflict Resolution.
Bandura, A. (1977). *Social Learning Theory.* Englewood Cliffs, NJ: Prentice-Hall.
Bock, R., & English, A. (1973). *Got Me on the Run.* Boston: Beacon.

Brandon, J. S. & Folk, S. (1977). Runaway adolescents' perceptions of parents and self. *Adolescence, 12*, 175-187.

Brennan, T., Huizinga, D., & Elliott, D. S. (1978). *The Social Psychology of Runaways.* Lexington, MA: D. C. Heath.

Cowen, E. & Work, W. (1988). Resilient children, psychological wellness, and primary prevention. *American Journal of Community Psychology, 16,* 591-607.

Gordon, T. (1975). *Parent Effectiveness Training: Instructor's Manual.* Solana Beach, CA: Sage.

Hepsworth, D. H., & Larsen, J. (1986). *Direct Social Work Practice: Theory and Skills* (2nd ed.). Chicago: Dorsey Press.

Hildebrand, J. A. (1968). Reasons for runaways. *Crime and Delinquency,* 14(1): 42-48.

Howing, P. T., Hawkins, J. D., Lishner, D. M., Catalano, R. F., & Howard, M. O. (1986). Childhood predictions of adolescent substance abuse: Toward an empirically grounded theory. *Journal of Children in Contemporary Society,* 8, 11-48.

Morrison, M. A. (1985).Adolescence and vulnerability to chemical dependencey. *Insight 1,* Atlanta, GA: Ridgeview Institute.

National Institute on Alcohol Abuse and Alcoholism (1986). *Helping your child say "NO" to alcohol.* (1986). Washington, DC: Office of Substance Abuse, Department of Health and Human Services, Public Health Services, Alcohol Drug Addiction and Mental Health Administration.

Patterson, G. R. & Forgatch, M. S. (1987). *Parents and Adolescents Living Together. Part 1: The Basics.* Eugene, OR: Castalia.

Robin, A. L. & Foster, S. L. (1989). Negotiating parent-adolescent conflict: A behavioral family systems approach. *Behavior Therapist,* 13(3):69.

Robinson, P. A. (1978). Parents of "beyond control" adolescents. *Adolescence,* 13(49):109-119.

Suddick, D. (1973). Runaways: A review of the literature. *Juvenile Justice,* 24:46-54.

Vandeloo, M. C. (1977). A study of coping behavior of runaway adolescents as related to situational stresses. *Dissertation Abstracts International,* 38:2387-2388B. (University Microfilms No. 5-B).

Williams, R. L., & Long, J. D. (1979). *Toward a Self-Managed Lifestyle.* Boston: Houghton Mifflin Co.

Wodarski, J. S. (1987a). *Adolescent depression and suicide prevention: Instructor's training manual for parent component.* Unpublished manuscript. The University of Georgia School of Social Work, Athens.

Wodarski, J. S. (1987b). Evaluating a social learning approach to teaching adolescents about alcohol and driving: A multiple variable evaluation. *Journal of Social Science Research, 10,* 121-144.

Wodarski, J. S. & Thyer, B. A. (1989). Behavioral perspectives on the family: An overview. In *Behavioral Family Interventions,* ed. Thyer, B. (Ed.). Springfield, IL: Charles C. Thomas.

Wodarski, J. S. & Wodarski, L. A. (1993). *Curriculums and Practical Aspects of Implementation: Preventive Health Services for Adolescents.* Lanham, MD: University Press of America, Inc.

Vender Zanden, J. W. (1978). *Human development.* New York: Alfred A. Knopf.

Zastrow, C. & Kirst-Ashman, K. (1987). *Understanding Human Behavior And The Social Environment.* Chicago: Nelson-Hall Publishers.

Chapter 5

The Alteration of Adolescent Substance Abuse: A Macro-Level Approach

America today is a chemical culture. For example, in Georgia, a state with a population of 6 million people, one billion dollars were spent in 1982 on alcohol and drugs, and 60 billion dollars were spent in the United States (Morrison, 1985). The use and abuse of chemical substances exacts an incalculable cost for substance abusers and non-substance abusers alike. Drug abuse-related deaths, injury, disease, and family and emotional disturbance are consequences that cannot be measured in monetary figures (Gallegos & Morrison, 1987). Annually, 100,000 to 120,000 deaths are directly attributable to substance abuse, and another 120,000 to 150,000 deaths are substance abuse-related (Gallegos & Morrison, 1987). Even more alarming, in 1988, 6 percent of 12- to 17-year-olds consumed alcohol daily, 4 percent used marijuana daily, and 0.5 percent used cocaine daily (American Medical Association, 1991).

Adolescence is a time of growth, stress, and change. This developmental stage affects not only the adolescent but his or her family as well. Adolescents, while in the natural process of establishing autonomy and identity, begin to separate from parents and experiment with a variety of behaviors and lifestyle patterns (Botvin, 1983). It is during adolescence when the relative importance of family and peers begins to shift. The peer group becomes more central for the adolescent, and the adolescent begins to rely more heavily on peers for support, security, and guidance (Belsky, Lerner, & Spanier, 1984; Kandel and Davies, 1991). Establishing peer relationships and peer acceptance are the hallmarks of adolescence; and the need to gain acceptance, approval, and praise is greater during adolescence than at any other time in life (Morrison, 1985).

193

Many adolescents experience confusion and turmoil as they strive to achieve autonomy. Because of the experienced turmoil and confusion, adolescents often perceive taking psychoactive substances as one of their few pleasurable options (Morrison & Smith, 1987). According to Morrison (1985) the use and abuse of mood altering chemical substances is now an integral part of growing into adulthood in the United States. Morrison (1985) notes that two-thirds of high school students use drugs and alcohol with regular frequency, and 85 percent of these students use drugs and alcohol at least three times a week. Additionally, 65 percent to 70 percent of junior high school students use drugs and alcohol two to three times weekly (Morrison, 1985).

When one adds tobacco and alcohol and other legal drugs the figures are staggering. The amount of alcohol and tobacco consumed by adolescents is enormous. The economic loss is difficult to assess because it is not clear how much time is missed from school and/or work. However, adolescence is usually the period when tobacco and alcohol use is developed. The formation and consequences of long-term problems take place after adolescence. One major consequence of alcohol use in adolescence is with driving. The evidence is clear that drinking and driving is a terrible mix with the consequences of death and injuries becoming almost routine.

There are other consequences of tobacco and alcohol abuse for which the adolescent may be a victim. Parental drinking problems affect adolescents because they are apt to be affected by a wide range of social problems. For example, alcohol use has been implicated in incest, child abuse, child neglect, rape, and a host of other violent crimes. Smoking may shorten the life of a parent or increase the severity of certain childhood diseases, such as asthma. Thus, adolescents are likely to be affected directly by exposure to alcohol and tobacco usage of their parents and others, often before they begin to show the effects of their own usage. It is important to recognize that alcohol is normally the drug that starts the cycle of drug use in our society. The myth that marijuana is the gateway drug leading to use of more serious drugs such as heroin and cocaine is inaccurate. However, alcohol has been identified as the drug of choice first used by pre-adolescents.

Youth are making decisions about the role alcohol and drugs will play in their lives. This is a timely, large-looming decision every adolescent must face; hence, there is a crucial need for teenagers to have an accurate, broad, well-rounded foundation of knowledge to draw upon when making decisions about alcohol and drug use.

Most often, the contact point of visibility of adolescents facing alcohol and drug issues is the school setting where adolescents spend approximately 50 percent of their waking hours. School composes the society of youth–in this arena parents are excluded; the rulers are peers, with teachers at best playing the role of consultants. The greater the amount of quality time teachers and administrators devote to substance abuse education to assist adolescents in learning self-management skills related to substance use, the greater the likelihood of insuring against a haphazard, hit-or-miss approach to adolescents' life decisions pertaining to substance use and abuse.

Effective comprehensive methods of teaching youth about psychoactive substances are imperative if they are to make well-informed decisions about their use (Ellickson & Bell, 1990). In order to fully impact on youth, the most critical point for receptivity seems to be the early adolescent years–following the influence of the parental/home setting and coinciding with the influx of peer influence. If the peer group is met successfully with a sociocultural approach to change the social norms surrounding substance use, then peers can make knowledgeable, unpressured, individual decisions regarding the use of psychoactive substances.

Macro level variables that might be altered to prevent substance abuse among teenagers are discussed. This chapter reviews the following sub-macro level systems: school and peer environment, home and family, community movements, and business and industry in terms of how they can be employed to prevent abuse among teenagers. The chapter concludes with an elucidation of what must be done to influence youths' drug behaviors.

SCHOOL AND PEER GROUP ENVIRONMENT

Youth spend the majority of their lives in the school setting. The school system, therefore, seems to be a natural forum for implementation of change. Educational programs aimed at prevention and early intervention can instill socially acceptable and responsible guidelines for drinking as well as for other problem behaviors (Dembo, Farrow, Schmeidler, & Burgos, 1979; Ellickson and Bell, 1990; Gottfredson 1986 & 1988; Gottfredson, & Cook, 1986).

Irresponsible drug use by teens takes its toll in other ways also. The abusing teen may feel isolated from nonabusing peers. Crime may become a factor to deal with when the adolescent has to steal to maintain drug habits. There are also developmental issues to be recognized. Adolescents already dealing with stressful changes in their lives may compound the stress with drug abuse. They are changing in physical, emotional, and sexual ways and must deal with new roles, feelings, and identities.

The issue is further compounded by multiple abuse patterns. Young people frequently use alcohol in combination with other drugs, principally marijuana (Lowman et al., 1982; Turanski, 1983). This combination of alcohol and drugs adds to the difficulty in treating youths and their changing values.

The ideal program should have two foci. First, the information transmission approach to provide basic knowledge and awareness, and second, the responsible decision approach that will teach youngsters the basic coping and decision-making skills (Schinke & Gilchrist, 1984).

Programs must take advantage of peer pressure in a positive manner. To be nonjudgmental and to develop self-esteem in these vulnerable youths are goals of utmost importance and urgency. In program planning there is a need for youth to provide input regarding what they feel are their greatest stresses; programs need to directly address these issues.

Many youths use drugs as a coping mechanism. School pressures and adolescent growth (both emotional and physical) are all basic life problems. The schools can offer meaningful alternatives to drugs to help adolescents deal with these stressors. A variety of activities can be offered by schools to provide teenagers reinforcements other than drugs. These after-school programs will be successful when they center on youths' interests such as music, fashion, sports, and so forth. For example, gyms can be kept open on weekends and during summer months, a small price compared to the effects of substance abuse.

The problem in reaching these adolescents comes when they do not see their drug use as a problem but as a regular boredom-relieving activity. "When alcohol-using youth are asked if they see their alcohol use as a problem . . . the most frequently encountered reply is 'no'" (Turanski, 1983, p. 4). When they do recognize a problem, youth are ill-prepared to seek help. They are more often than not unaware of prevention and treatment centers. Moreover, they may view these services with mistrust, fear, and embarrassment. Another great fear is exposure to both parents and the law. Thus, communication has to occur regarding services that are available. Service providers have to reach out to the youths who are at risk.

To date little emphasis has been placed in educational settings on teenage alcohol use and its subsequent effect on driving (Wodarski & Hoffman, 1984). An innovative program with documented success is the "Alcohol Education by Teams-Games-Tournaments" approach.

"Teams-Games-Tournaments" (TGT) is another educational approach aimed at teaching youths, through noncompetitive games, to learn self-management skills and facts about drugs through behavioral analysis (Lenhart & Wodarski, 1983). The goal of the TGT technique is to assist teenagers in making decisions to drink or abstain, how to drink, how often and how much, and to foster the attitude of responsible drinking. The TGT approach is realistic. Its aim is to teach awareness and responsibility and not to proselytize prohibition and abstinence. The uniqueness of TGT is that it capitalizes on peers as teachers to aid in the acquisition of knowledge about drugs and their effects on behavior.

Subsequent research has developed the Comprehensive Psychoactive Substance Use Education Program for Adolescents. It is targeted to provide essential knowledge to adolescents about psychoactive substances in such a manner as to be a fun, peer group experience, thus increasing the likelihood of acquisition of knowledge and behavior. The program is comprised of three parts: education about psychoactive substance, self-management skills related to substance use, and the maintenance of knowledge and behavior. The instructional method of the comprehensive program is the Teams-Games-Tournaments (TGT) technique.

Before beginning the education phase of the program, students are assessed for level of psychoactive substance knowledge. The completion of the pretest of psychoactive substance knowledge will provide the basis for division of students into four-member teams. The teams will be organized into high achievers (those with a high level of psychoactive substance knowledge), middle achievers (those with moderate levels), and low achievers (those most lacking in psychoactive substance knowledge). Team composition will be heterogeneous, with one high achiever, two middle achievers and one low achiever on each team, so that the average achievement level will be approximately equal across teams.

Behavioral analysis over the last 15 years has been applied to the solution of many classroom problems, including discipline and the teaching of verbal, reading, and arithmetic skills. This is the first curriculum study in a pilot effort to teach substance abuse education to secondary students through behavioral analysis. TGT is preferred over individual classroom instruction substance abuse education for several reasons. First, the group learning situation most closely resembles the setting in which adolescents make their decisions regarding the use of substances among peers. And since substance abuse most often takes place in group settings, knowledge acquired in the group setting is more likely to be used when in similar peer group settings than knowledge acquired through individual, separate means (Allman, Taylor, & Nathan, 1972; Feldman & Wodarski, 1975; Wodarski & Bagarozzi, 1979). From the perspective of the educator, the group method allows for a broader range of learning experience; students have the opportunity to learn while interacting with peers in a friendly, exciting game. Refer to Chapter 3 for comprehensive discussion of the TGT method.

The psychoactive substance use education units provided in this guide are to be presented for fifty minutes each day for six weeks. The first three days of each week are to be devoted to learning the psychoactive substance concepts in the exercises, discussions, and various participatory activities. The fourth day is to be focused on working in the TGT teams on worksheets in preparation for the tournament which is to be held on the fifth day of each week.

THE FAMILY

Young people need positive role models from which to gain their experiences. Data indicate that adolescents are more likely to consume alcohol in a manner similar to that of their parents (Wodarski & Hoffman, 1984) and the parents' drinking behavior is an important influence (Bacon & Jones, 1968).

One of the most devastating aspects of alcohol use is that children are very likely to be introduced to alcohol by their parents, friends, or family members. Beer is usually the favorite drug and children, sometimes as young as eight, are introduced to the culture by those close to them.

In regard to the family, we have noted that alcohol is the first drug to which children are normally introduced, and they tend to develop drinking habits in preadolescence and then accelerate them in their adolescent phase. During this period large amounts of beer and other, stronger drinks are likely to be consumed. In college, it is frequently noted that almost 90-95 percent of the students have consumed alcohol. Many continue to drink alcohol regularly during their college years. Indeed alcohol remains the drug of choice for students in college as well as in high school, far in advance of all the other drugs combined.

It is quite evident that the family plays a crucial part in the formation of habits and attitudes regarding drug use. The consuming of pills at an early age, the taking of medicine to make one feel well, watching Mommy or Daddy take different colored pills to get rid of pain, provides youngsters with the idea that drugs are an excellent way to make one feel better. Without any discussion in the family where drugs are used, whether they be aspirin, other over-the-counter drugs, legal or illegal drugs, youngsters are very likely to learn that it is all right to use drugs because they make one feel better, relieve stress and tension, and make one's problems and difficulties go away.

The family is the "crucial influence on children's values and behavior" (Lieberman, Caroff, & Gottesfeld, 1973). In the home, youth can find structure and guidance from loved ones who really care about them. Clear expectations about consumption can be communicated. Younger children are especially vulnerable to pressures and they need a trusting and comfortable place to turn for help in mastering their anxieties and frustrations. The home is the stabilizing influence for youth. It should be the place to turn where alcohol-induced states are not glorified.

Parents must realize that in regard to alcohol and driving they maintain ultimate control. Parents are the resource for the car availability. Mom and Dad have the power to keep abusing adolescents from using the car. Parents need to be reinforced that they have the responsibility and right to make decisions that are in the best interests of their children.

Parents may need help in asserting themselves and in coping with difficult situations. Support is available through such mechanisms as Parent Effectiveness Training (PET) classes where parents learn better parenting skills. Through such training, parents learn to set clear expectations about drinking and to enforce consequences when expectations are not met. Moreover, they practice ways to open lines of communication to discuss the use of alcohol and its effects with their teenager.

MEDIA

The media exert a powerful influence on contemporary society. Examples of both positive and negative portrayals of drinking behavior are aired throughout the viewing period. Depending on the programming, the messages are as varied as "drinking is mandated for a good time" and "to be a good friend, do not let your friend drink and drive." Young people watch television and see the message of what they need and what they should want. "Tuning in can lead to turning off by turning on" (Lieberman et al., 1973, p. 110). Also, as Globetti (1977) suggests, "adolescents . . . view alcohol mostly in terms of sociability and in the sense of what it does for them rather than to them."

The significant impact of daytime and nighttime T.V. "soaps" needs to be evaluated. Many programs need parental interpretation. Excessive consumption of alcohol as portrayed in these shows is equated with power and success. In reality adolescents must be informed that such consumption more likely impedes success.

The media can likewise exert a powerful positive influence. One of the favorite pastimes of contemporary youth is music. The messages this media conveys must be considered since it is a continual influence. Positive role models affect the norms of youth and must be capitalized upon. Rather than glorify the consumption of drugs and its association with adventure and sex, role models can "turn on" teens to more positive outlets.

The media is an extremely important component in a macro approach to substance abuse. The media is in a position to place or exert a powerful positive or negative influence on all people, particularly adolescents. Each substance abuse class led by one of the authors over the past several years compiled a survey of substance abuse articles which appeared in their local newspaper. An analysis of the newspaper accounts in each year led to a conclusion that drugs, particularly illicit drugs, are an African-American problem. This myth was perpetuated by the inclusion of a picture, often on page one, of a drug abuser or of police apprehending a drug offender who was African American. The evidence was that the overwhelming majority of pictures that appeared in the local newspaper during these several years were of African Americans, usually males (Harrison, Nodarski, & Thyer, 1992).

Such media images do not portray the seriousness of the problem nor do they accurately reflect the extent of the substance abuse problem in this country. Data reveal that over 75 percent of the substance abusers in this country are white and that in fact drug use among African-American adolescents tends to be lower than that of other racial or ethnic group counterparts. Yet this image of illicit drug use being an African-American problem continues to be portrayed in the media.

The point to the exercise was to demonstrate the powerful effect that media has upon the public. Thus, one of the more effective ways of dealing with the public would be to encourage the media to present more accurate and more factual information about the problem of substance abuse in our community, rather than projecting what they think the public wants to hear or see and then disseminating a negative image of particular populations.

COMMUNITY MOVEMENTS

The ability to influence community norms rests within the community itself. By joining forces and establishing coalitions, standards of acceptance of drinking and driving under the influence of alcohol can be changed (Blansfield, 1984; Gardner, 1983).

Community efforts are an excellent way of dealing with substance abuse problems in the community. A major difficulty with local efforts is that they must be maintained over long periods of time to be effective. Community efforts also involve great cost and personal involvement of key people in the area who have a strong desire to have drugs removed from their locality.

However, often lacking is the continued long-term effort needed to rid the communities of the drug pushers and drug users. The drug dealers and users usually move to other locations and keep rotating or moving in order to keep ahead of community efforts and police action. Consider this scenario: as a community becomes effective in dealing with the substance abuse problem, the drug dealers, pushers, and users all move to another location. The community program participants consider their effort quite successful and may continue their vigil over a reasonable period of time. However, the drug dealers and users keep moving to other locations, and it takes considerable time before local people realize what is happening. Thus, while one community is keeping pace and trying to rid itself of drug dealers and users, another community program, considered successful, begins to disband. Thus, you have a rotating effect wherein one community becomes successful and disbands its program, but yet another area has become infected. This cycle is repeated often. Thus, while community efforts can be excellent and effective, the need for continued support by law enforcement personnel, and the need to maintain a vigilant effort over extremely long periods of time renders this approach uneven (Walker, 1989).

LAWS AND ENFORCEMENT

Individual and community involvement and pressure can result in significant social change through governmental legislation and policy (Pentz, Brannon, Charlin, Barrett, MacKinnon, & Flay, 1989). Public law can have either a positive or a negative effect, depending on enforcement. An example of a law that has had a positive effect is the raising of the legal drinking age to 21, as it has reduced the death rate in the 18-21 year old age group. It is impor-

tant to note that uniform enforcement of this law still remains difficult to achieve, however, by raising the drinking age to 21 years the
overall effect has been to reduce the accessibility of alcohol available to the under 21 population. Reduced accessibility particularly
on campuses and court action holding families and owners of tav-
erns liable for serving alcohol to impaired individuals has served to
decrease the incidents of drinking and driving in our communities.

However, enforcement is not an easy answer to drug problems in
our communities. Existing laws and their uneven enforcement re-
main a crazy patchwork making fairness and justice very obscure.
Moreover, the outcomes of enforcement are often unclear. For example, in the years 1980-1992 it has been estimated that 70 percent
of all drug dollars went to law enforcement. Yet by all accounts the
availability of drugs in our communities has not abated significant-
ly, and, in fact, there appears to be more drugs available today than
ever before. Therefore, it is not very clear what law enforcement
activities had upon the overall availability of drugs.

While surveys indicate that overall drug usage may have decreased, it is also clear that the types of drugs consumed shift over
time. A good example of this shift in usage occurs when pressure is
applied by law enforcement agencies to curtail certain illicit drugs.
Dealers and users tend to shift to other drugs not under surveillance.

One of the reasons enforcement is difficult is that one must
recognize that drug availability is a market commodity. Therefore,
drugs are made available by pushers and purchased by the consumer as any other product. Thus, when one drug becomes difficult for
the consumer to buy or for the pusher to have available, the price of
the drug will naturally rise. When this occurs other drugs become
available at a more reasonable price.

There are also some serious problems with drug sentencing. It
would appear that at best drug sentencing is applied deferentially
such that in certain states drug offenses may be viewed more liber-
ally whereas in other states the same offense can be dealt with rather
harshly. For example, an individual may be apprehended and convicted with a small amount of the drug in his or her possession, and
may receive a harsher penalty than someone who commits a second
degree murder or who has committed a violent crime. Thus, the
sentencing guidelines and the types of sentences that people who

are convicted of drug offenses receive are usually disproportionate to the seriousness of the offense. The outcome is that a vast majority of the people in prisons have drug-related offenses while other crimes and perhaps more serious offenses in our society are being treated less harshly.

On a more interesting note it remains odd that there are severe penalties for illicit drugs such as heroin, cocaine, and marijuana. However, many other drugs are legal including alcohol, tobacco, amphetamines, barbiturates, and many over-the-counter drugs which are consumed daily. It should be noted that almost 25 years ago the Federal government made methadone legal. A whole treatment system was legalized for a drug which is more addicting than heroin. This drug was made available to many heroin addicts at a very low cost with the population being treated under medical supervision and government control; this policy continues to the present.

It is, therefore, difficult to understand the position of people who do not want to make drugs legal. The solution implies not only the reduction of crime by pricing drugs at reasonable cost to the consumer, but it also reduces the rather harsh penalties given to people who are involved with only a select few drugs. This selectivity of penalties for certain drugs, which tend not to be the most injurious to an individual's health, remains very confusing to many people. Another example of the confusing legal structure of penalties in this field is that marijuana is classed a schedule one drug: i.e., one with no medicinal value and a high potential of addiction. Yet marijuana is not considered addicting by the medical community (although government brochures say it may be addicting), and alcohol produces the most toxic effects on one's body of all drugs. Yet alcohol is not even mentioned on the schedule of drugs.

To explain the rationale behind the schedule of drugs and the determination of drugs which are illicit and licit often defies logic and credibility. Until our society determines a sensible approach to all drugs there will not be any effective and long-term solution to the drug abuse problem in our country. Complicating any resolution of the drug problem in our country is the fact that this is a drug-taking and a drug-consuming society. There is virtually no distinction between the drugs, including alcohol, children witness their parents consume until the time they are old enough to start consuming a variety of pills and drugs on their own, and the incredible number of drugs made available to them through the medical and dental communities and through advertisements. In short, there remains a huge consuming population for which the often-stated goal of a drug-free society is entirely illusory. It remains useful for only a few zealots and for those who continue to invest heavily in a punitive and law enforcement approach. Clearly the time has come for this nation to rethink and recast its societal approach to drug usage (Kappler, Blumberg, & Potter, 1993; MacCoun, 1993).

BUSINESS AND INDUSTRY

Business and industry have shown concern about irresponsible drinking and driving under the influence of alcohol. They have been spurred to action by data that indicate that productivity is substantially reduced when workers drink excessively (Mayer, 1983). Moreover, they are recognizing that work is a central aspect in many lives and supportive business can foster positive attitudes concerning the consumption of alcohol. Their commitment has been expressed by repeated advertisements in the media. They are reaching a large number of markets through use of print media, such as advertisements in major magazines. Business sponsored radio and television spots also promote responsible drinking. These spots have been used especially during holiday periods when people of all ages celebrate by irresponsibly using alcohol.

A General Motors advertisement that explains blood alcohol concentrations begins with a disclaimer: "First, you should understand that drinking any amount of alcohol can impair your ability to drive" (General Motors, 1983). The advertisement copy goes on to explain that General Motors has developed a device to test drivers' reflexes and responses before it allows the car to start. The Department of Transportation in California is now testing the device as a deterrent to repeat offenders. General Motors has made other commitments. For example, it set up a program for alcohol abuse in 1972 and it has expanded its Employee Assistance Program to include every General Motors installation in the United States and 12 that are located in Canada.

ISSUES

Family Intervention

Data indicate that parents whose adolescents are at risk face multiple social and psychological difficulties (Labouvie & McGee, 1986). The clearest empirical finding with regard to adolescents at risk seems to be the lack of consistency by the parent or parents in the handling of their children and the consequent lack of effectiveness in managing the child's behavior in a manner that facilitates his or her psychological and social development. It has also been pointed out that another common feature of relationships between parents and adolescents at risk is unrealistic expectations by the parents regarding what is appropriate behavior for their child (Howing, Wodarski, Kurtz & Gaudin, 1989; Patterson & Forgatch, 1987; Wodarski & Thyer, 1989).

Another empirical finding of substance has been the high degree of strain evident in families with children at risk. Family interaction patterns have been characterized as primarily negative; that is, parents engage in excessive amounts of criticism, threats, negative statements, physical punishment, and a corresponding lack of positive interaction such as positive statements, praise, positive physical contact, and so forth (Zigler, Taussig, & Black, 1992). In view of this finding, a comprehensive prevention approach should include appropriate interventions that teach knowledge about the problems adolescents face, communication skills, problem solving, and conflict resolution to family members. Each intervention package must have an attractive and effective parent curriculum.

Timing of the Intervention

Recent research executed on various populations indicated that intervention should occur in the fourth, fifth, and sixth grades to psychologically inoculate children for the risks that they are going to face. All of the interventions discussed within this manuscript should be executed as early as possible. Ideally, booster sessions would occur as children move into junior high and high school. These booster sessions should include procedures for the maintenance and generalization of behaviors such as: training relatives or significant others in the child's environment; training behaviors that have a high probability of being reinforced in natural environments; varying the conditions of training; gradually removing or fading the contingencies; using different schedules of reinforcement; using delayed reinforcement and self-control procedures (Wodarski & Wodarski, 1993).

Curriculum

Updates should occur periodically. Material that is included in the curriculum should be easily comprehended and presented in an attractive manner. All updates should include information that is relevant for the skills that are being acquired. Moreover, role playing exercises which involve overlearning should be included. Such exercises make up the requisites of relevant curriculums. The social skills training paradigm offers social workers an excellent procedure for preparing adolescents to live successfully in contemporary American society. The curriculums are particularly relevant to social group work since data indicate that peers play a strong role in the acquisition of either social or dysfunctional behaviors. The small group learning techniques that are elucidated within the manuscript capitalize on peers as teachers. Thus, social workers are provided with viable techniques that can capitalize on peer structures to help adolescents acquire necessary social behaviors to deal competently with the requisites of adolescent development.

CONCLUSION

The solution to the problem of drug consumption among teens requires an all-out effort by those societal forces capable of effecting change. Families, schools, peers, communities, businesses, and the media all possess powers to eradicate this social problem. The campaign cannot be waged from only one front, however. Combined, cooperative efforts are essential. The responsibility must be shared for both the prior condoning of actions that have perpetuated the problem and for working toward mutual goals and solutions.

REFERENCES

Alcohol Health and Research World, March 3, 1983.

Allman, R., Taylor, H. A., & Nathan, P. E. (1972). Group drinking during stress: Effects on drinking behavior, affect, and psychopathology. *American Journal of Psychiatry* 129(6):45-54.

American Medical Association (1991). *Profiles of Adolescent Health.* Vol. 2. Adolescent Health Care: Use, Costs, and Problems of Access.

Bacon, M. & Jones, M. B. (1968). *Teenage Drinking.* New York: Thomas Y. Crowell Company.

Belsky, K. J., Lerner, R. M., & Spanier, G. B. (1984). *The Child in the Family.* New York: Random House.

Blansfield, H.N. (1984). Drinking and/or driving. *Connecticut Medicine,* 48(3), 205.

Botvin, G. J. (1983). Prevention of adolescent substance abuse through the development of personal and social competence. In *Preventing Adolescent Drug Abuse: Intervention Strategies,* Glynn, T., Surkefeld, C., & Sudford, J. (Eds.). (DHHS Publication No. ADM 83-1280). Washington, DC: U.S. Government Printing Office.

Dembo, R., Farrow, D., Schmeidler, J., & Burgos, W. (1979). Testing a causal model of environmental influences on early drug involvement of inner city junior high school youths. *American Journal of Drug and Alcohol Abuse,* 6, 313-336.

Ellickson, P. L. & Bell, R. M. (1990). Drug prevention in junior high: A multi-site longitudinal test. *Science* 247:1299-1305.

Feldman, R. A. & Wodarksi, J. S. (1975). *Contemporary Approaches to Group Treatment.* San Francisco: Jossey-Bass.

Gallegos, K. V. & Morrison, M. A. (1987). *Substance Abuse Adolescents: Implications for the Year 2000.*

Gardner, S.E. (1983). *Communities: What you can do about drug and alcohol abuse* (DHHS Pub. No. ADM-84-1310). Rockville, MD: National Institute on Drug Abuse.

General Motors, July 1983, 5. Customer information from General Motors. GEO, (advertisement).

Globetti, G. (1977). Teenage drinking. In *Alcoholism: Development, Consequences and Interventions.* N. J. Estes and M. E. Heinemann (Eds.). St. Louis: C. V. Mosby Company.

Gottfredson, D. C. (1986). An empirical test of school-based environmental and individual interventions to reduce the risk of delinquent behavior. *Criminology,* 24, 705-731.

Gottfredson, D. C. (1988). An evaluation of an organization development approach to reducing school disorder. *Evaluation Review*, 11, 739-763.

Gottfredson, D. C., & Cook, M. S. (1986). *Increasing school relevance and student decision making: Effective strategies for reducing delinquency?* Unpublished manuscript, Johns Hopkins University, Center for the Social Organization of Schools, Baltimore.

Harrison, D., Wodarski, J.S., & Thyer, B. (1992). *Cultural Diversity and Social Work Practice,* Springfield, IL: Charles C. Thomas.

Howing, P. T., Wodarski, J. S., Kurtz, D. P., & Gaudin, J. M. (1990). The empirical base for the implementation of social skills training with maltreated children. *Social Work*, Vol. 35(5), p.460-467.

Kandel, D. B. & Davies, M. (1991). Cocaine use in a national sample of U.S. youth (NLSY): Epidemiology, predictors, and ethnic patterns. In *The Epidemiology of Cocaine Use and Abuse* (NIDA research monograph, DHHS Publication No. ADM 91-1787, pp. 151-188). Washington, DC: U.S. Government Printing Office.

Kappler, V. E., Blumberg, M., & Potter, G. W. (1993). *The Mythology of Crime and Criminal Justice.* Prospect Heights, IL: Waveland Press, Inc.

Labouvie, E. W., & McGee, C. R. (1986). Relation of personality to alcohol and drug use in adolescence. *Journal of Consulting and Clinical Psychology*, 54, 289-293.

Lenhart, S. D., & Wodarski, J. S. (1983). *Alcohol Education by the Teams-Games-Tournaments Method* (2nd ed.). Minneapolis, MN: Alpha Editions.

Lieberman, F., Caroff, P., & Gottesfeld, M. (1973). *Before Addiction: How to Help Youth.* New York: Behavioral Publications.

Lowman, C., Hubbard, R. L., Rachal, J. V., & Cavanaugh, E. R. (1982). Facts for planning: Adolescent marijuana and alcohol use. *Alcohol Health and Research World*, 6(3), 69-75.

MacCoun, R. J. (1993). Drugs and the law: A psychological analysis of drug prohibition. *Psychological Bulletin, 113*(3), 497-512.

Mayer, W. (1983). Alcohol abuse and alcoholism: The psychologist's role in prevention, research, and treatment. *American Psychologist, 38*(10), 1116-1121.

Morrison, M. A. (1985). Adolescence and vulnerability to chemical dependence. *Insight,* 1, Atlanta, GA: Ridgeview Institute.

Morrison, M. A. & Smith, T. Q. (1987). Psychiatric issues of adolescent chemical dependence. *Pediatric Clinics of North America, 34*(2):461-480.

Patterson, G. R., & Forgatch, M. S. (1987). *Parents and Adolescents Living Together. Part 1: The Basics.* Eugene, OR: Castalia.

Pentz, M. A., Brannon, B. R., Charlin, V. L., Barrett, E. J., MacKinnon, D. P., & Flay, B. R. (1989). The power of policy: Relationship of smoking policy to adolescent smoking. *American Journal of Public Health*, 79, 857-862.

Schinke, S. P. & Gilchrist, L. D. (1984). *Life Skills Counseling with Adolescents.* Baltimore: University Park Press.

Turanski, J. J. (1983). Reaching and treating youth with alcohol-related problems: A comprehensive approach. *Alcohol, Health and Research World,* 7(4), 3-9.

Walker, S. (1989). *Sense and Nonsense about Crime,* 2nd Edition. Pacific Grove, CA: Brooks/Cole.

Wodarski, J. S. & Bagarozzi, D. (1979). *Behavioral Social Work.* New York: Human Sciences Press.

Wodarski, J. S. & Thyer, B. A. (1989). Behavioral perspectives on the family: An overview. In *Behavioral Family Interventions,* B. Thyer (Ed.). Springfield, IL: Charles C. Thomas.

Wodarski, J. S. & Wodarski, L. A. (1993). *Curriculums and Practical Aspects of Implementation: Preventive Health Services for Adolescents.* Lanham, MD: University Press of America, Inc.

Wodarski, J. S., & Hoffman, S. D. (1984). Alcohol education for adolescents. *Social Work in Education,* 6(2), 69-92.

Zigler, E., Taussig, C., & Black, K. (1992). Early childhood intervention: A promising preventive for juvenile delinquency. *American Psychologist, 47*(8), 997-1006.

Index